Thanks
for
Coming

HARPER ⬤ PERENNIAL

NEW YORK • LONDON • TORONTO • SYDNEY • NEW DELHI • AUCKLAND

Thanks for Coming

ONE YOUNG WOMAN'S QUEST FOR AN ORGASM

mara altman

For my parents

HARPER ● PERENNIAL

The names and identifying characteristics of some of the individuals featured throughout this book have been changed to protect their privacy.

P.S.™ is a trademark of HarperCollins Publishers.

HarperCollins books may be purchased for educational, business, or sales promotional use. For information please write: Special Markets Department, HarperCollins Publishers, 10 East 53rd Street, New York, NY 10022.

FIRST EDITION

Designed by Justin Dodd

Library of Congress Cataloging-in-Publication Data is available upon request.

ISBN 978-0-06-157711-6

09 10 11 12 13 OV/RRD 10 9 8 7 6 5 4 3 2 1

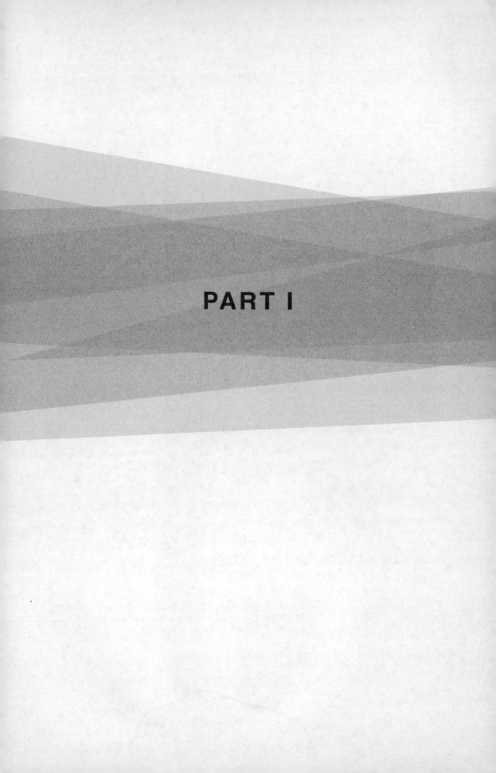

PART I

WHERE'S THE KEY TO MY CLI-TAURUS?

I called up Dr. Barry Komisaruk. "No orgasm!?" he said when I told him that my orgasm gear—all that stuff "down there"—was out of whack. He must have heard the urgency in my voice, because the New Jersey–based neuroscientist said he'd meet me in the City. But before hanging up the phone, he started taking down notes. "How old are you? You have siblings? Have you tried . . ."

Dr. Komisaruk had recently published a book, *The Science of Orgasm*, with two coauthors. He seemed to know everything about the subject, and I was hoping he could help me out since nothing I had tried so far was working. Of course, an essential, yet quite counterproductive, part of my problem was that "trying" didn't actually include me touching myself.

But more on that later.

See, I'm twenty-six years old and don't have one climax to show for it. Even the three cats—Buddy, Sika, and Lucy—running around my Brooklyn apartment manage to remind me of that fact. They upchuck, lick themselves, claw at things, and hump each other in front of me, and I wonder how we humans, especially me, got so far away from the instinctual. My instincts seem kaput; they atrophied because I wasn't exercising them regularly. I want to hump a sofa pillow and pat myself on the back for it—good girl!— but I haven't even been able to touch my crotch, let alone hump a pillow. I'm suffering from a case of inhibition, which might be compounded by some love cynicism.

I looked up the statistics. Forty-three percent of women report having some sort of sexual dysfunction, so I shouldn't be too horrified, but the more I think about my own problem, the more it freaks me out. When I gave a girlfriend of mine the news, she practically dropped to the curb like it was a pew and prayed for me—an especially dazzling performance given that she's an atheist.

Dr. Komisaruk agreed to meet me at an Indian restaurant on Bleecker Street in the Village. I suggested Ethiopian, but he said the last time he ate that cuisine, he got confused and used the flat rolls of bread to wipe the beads of sweat off his forehead. He thought it was a hot towel. It left an uncomfortable doughy feeling on his skin that he didn't want to relive. Neuroscientists can't be smart about everything.

It's not like I haven't had sex; I have, with six men. (Actually, let's call it five and a half, but more on that later.) But back to orgasms—or rather, lack of them. No, I haven't had one. An orgasm seems just as elusive with my own touch as it was with any of my five and a half men, and I want to fix that. I've managed to travel around the world—I've lived in Spain, India, Thailand, and Peru and had plenty of relationship casualties along the way—but I've never ventured inside myself. And so the journey I've decided to take—the one that led me to call Dr. Komisaruk—is going to be about stepping outside my comfort zone and pushing my own boundaries and ending my prudish ways. That's what I told myself anyway, but so far it's proving to be harder than I thought.

My project did not have an auspicious start. A few weeks ago, I'd set up an appointment with a sexologist named Melinda. I was an anxious mess as I entered her office. I was sweating like I'd crawled through a jungle—lagoons under my arms and eddies coalescing on my upper lip.

Melinda told me to get comfortable on her flower-print sofa. The sofa was the wrong fit. If I sat on the edge, my feet dangled, and if I sat all the way back, my legs stuck out like a toddler's in a minivan. Melinda couldn't talk to me about sex while I was sitting like that. It'd feel almost pedophilic. So I settled on Indian-style and tried to be Zen.

She resembled Bette Midler, but puffier. Conjure Midler clad in a football uniform but with longer hair, and instead of slinking around a stage singing about love, she's sitting on a sofa opposite and prodding *you* to sing about your embarrassing sexual hang-ups.

"I've never had an orgasm before," I said.

I began to elaborate on my theories—maybe I was rebelling against my parents, who are sex-loving hippies; maybe I was defining myself in contrast to my best friend, who lives on orgasms; maybe it could be the result of the Muslim guy I dated in India who didn't even know what a hand job was—but she cut me off and started educating me on what occurs in the body during arousal.

"The genitals get engorged with blood . . . throbbing."

"Hold up," I said. "Can we rewind?" I felt like I was on step 0.03 and she had galloped straight to ten.

"Just go home and touch your clitoris," she continued.

CLI-toris, is that how you say it? I've been saying cli-Taurus, like it was some kind of Ford sedan that needed to be started with a special key before I could take it for a spin around town.

WHERE'S THE KEY TO MY CLI-TAURUS?

Objectively, I knew I could just shove one of those rabbit vibrators everyone talks about down there and probably get it over with. But I didn't just see this as a physical issue: I wanted to know why, despite having been gifted many vibrators in my life, I hadn't attempted to use them yet.

To change the subject, I told her I was thinking about writing a book about the process. Before now, I had been so caught up in work, so obsessed with making something of myself, that it was entirely possible my pussy could have fallen off and I wouldn't have noticed. The only way I'd get in touch was if I made orgasm the focus of my work, made this odyssey part of my livelihood as a writer and journalist.

"That's a bad idea," she said.

In fact, she told me, writing about orgasm would be the absolute worst activity for someone who wanted to experience it.

"You can't think about orgasm," she said. "The more you ponder orgasm, the less likely you'll be to have one. You have to let go."

In other words, she was continuing her mantra: *Just touch the clit already!*

Melinda wouldn't budge; she reiterated her approach. "I'm straightforward," she said. "Is there a private place you feel comfortable touching yourself at home?"

I threw a pillow between my legs, guarding my groin, and shrugged. "My room has a door—is that what you mean?"

Our hour was up. When I went to use her bathroom, there were absolutely no traces of orgasm, only an old bar of soap and a flaky stick of deodorant. Trusting her would be like trusting a hairstylist who had a 'do like Ernie on *Sesame Street*. As she walked me to the door, she said she looked forward to working with me again but severely advised against writing: "You'll never orgasm if you think about it that much."

I couldn't take her advice to heart, somehow. Maybe it was the framed picture of the Vatican in her office. She seemed like the Anti-gasm.

From the Anti-gasm, I went to Google. I found an interesting Web site called Vulva University. It's run out of San Francisco. Dorrie Lane, the director, told me she was training the next generation of vulvalutionaries. Image evoked: the iconic red T-shirt with Che Guevara's black silhouette but replaced with a lone *mons pubis* wearing a beret. I wanted to be a vulvalutionary. Becoming a vulvalutionary almost seemed like a prerequisite for a girl who wanted to come, like me. Dorrie told me I could be one. All I needed was a vulva.

"Even a dysfunctional vagina?" I asked.

First she chided my genital semantics. She told me the word "vagina" only refers to the canal inside and accentuates only the female genitalia's penetrative capabilities, whereas "vulva," she said, includes all its various junk, such as the pleasure-inducing clit. She quickly went on to pitch her Wondrous Vulva Puppet, which she makes as a hobby. She said they are anatomically correct silk-lined twats. When you insert your hand, you can make the pussy talk by manipulating the labia minora as lips.

The stuffed vulvas were kind of cute, even though when I looked at the pictures online, they all looked more like extravagant catcher's mitts. That's probably why I liked them, actually, because when I checked out the other much more realistic vulvalutionary accessories—like the sterling silver vulva rings and necklace charms, which looked like elongated oysters with a pearl at the top deformed from a thorough dip in an acidic wash—I got a little skittish.

When my vulva puppet arrived—I'd ordered the model named Picchu, inspired by its colorful Peruvian tapestry-covered labia—

I'd expected it to help me verbalize some repressed and pent-up vaginal thoughts, like those of the real-open chicks who recite *The Vagina Monologues*, but that stuffed twat, which should have been my encouraging mascot, had nothing to say at all. It came in a silk drawstring bag. I hung it up forlornly on my doorknob.

And that's when I called up Dr. Komisaruk, distraught.

When we reach the restaurant, Dr. Komisaruk orders a bottle of wine, and as soon as he starts talking, I know he is my kind of man. He looks at me intently, and I can tell that orgasm isn't at all frivolous to him. He believes that every human being has the right to orgasm as strongly as Charlton Heston believed in the right to bear arms.

Dr. Komisaruk is in his sixties and has a calm pool of sun-spotted scalp on the crown of his head surrounded by crashing waves of gray hair. He wears standard khakis and a blue button-down dress shirt. He's on the cutting edge of orgasm research. He and his research partners throw women into fMRI machines, tell them to stimulate themselves, and then take pictures of where the orgasm sparks in their brains. Among other things, they've discovered that orgasm is a natural pain-blocker. While it lessens pain by up to fifty percent, the sensitivity of touch remains the same or even heightened, making a lover's caress all the sweeter.

I don't know if it is the spicy curries or the conversation that has me sweating, but it doesn't take long to get into the science of orgasms.

No one knows for sure why the female orgasm exists. Some contend that it's just evolutionary leftovers to the man's ejaculatory climax, like the male's little red nipples are to the female's milk-making mammaries. Others, such as Dr. Komisaruk, believe there's a purpose to a woman's flush-faced ecstasy, but he's not quite sure exactly what it is yet. It could be that the contractions of the uterus during orgasm help draw semen into the fallopian tubes to aid pregnancy, or that the pleasure tempts the woman to copulate again and again, or that orgasm allows a healthy release of muscle tension from the body—or it could be a mixture of all of the above.

Orgasmics tend to be less stressed than their non-orgasming counterparts, Dr. Komisaruk says.

"Barry," I say, practically falling into the curries, "do you think I'm stressed? I mean, really, do I look stressed to you?"

Dr. Komisaruk says he'd love to have me come over to his laboratory for an experiment. He'd have to wait for funding though; he says he's always waiting for funding.

"There's no premium on studying pleasure in this society," he explains.

He says when he gets the funding, he can put me in the fMRI machine and if I simultaneously watch my brain activity and prod myself with his stimulator, I could consciously try to activate the parts of my brain that usually light up during orgasm. Through biofeedback, I could cerebrally learn the response I am looking for, he says.

I tell him the closest thing I know to orgasm is the little tingle followed by a shudder I feel in the back of my neck when I clean my ears with Q-tips.

"Of course!" he says, as if he knows exactly what I am talking about. "An eargasm! But be careful, you can damage your ear canal."

"What?" I say, pretending I've already masturbated my ears to deaf.

He doesn't get my joke. "Careful! You have to be careful!" he warns.

He takes another piece of naan and dips it in his saag. To him, an orgasm is defined by a gradual buildup of tension, a peak, and then a release. He says many things can be a kind of orgasm: a sneeze, scratching an itch, laughing, crying, or even vomiting.

"It's a buildup of nausea and then . . ."

"Barry, that's not the kind of orgasm I'm looking for," I say.

I suddenly get that picture in my head of the orgasm I think I'm going to have one day: The material world disappears; it's been enveloped in a white light, similar to the one people always talk about at the end of the tunnel—tranquil yet inspiring you to draw near. In the absence of a view, a spectacular sunset transpires over my labial folds and sets behind my clitoral hood. I lose control of my body and forget where I am. If I were with someone, we'd both be suspended in time. This is where it gets weird. I turn into Scarlett Johansson. My little anti-knockers triple to three times their cup size and my back starts to arch. My pout opens just enough to bite off the tip of a chocolate-dipped strawberry, and all of a sudden the ruby-colored fruit is magically there. I think I'm slightly levitating by this point, and my skin glistens with this perfect layer of perspiration so that it almost sparkles like a lake at dawn, but not so much that the dew starts dripping. Then I start making all these really awesome sounds, kind of like the ones I make when I'm eating sashimi, but amplified and with a raspy cigarette-induced edge. I climax and it's like a sword of pleasure is puncturing my groin and every cell swells into a pool of transcendent bliss . . .

"Mara," says Dr. Komisaruk, "more navratan korma?"

"Oh," I say, "oh, yeah, sure."

I begin eating when Dr. Komisaruk divulges advice. "Do you have a vibrator?" he asks. "You need to get a powerful vibrator, that's what you need."

I drop the bread, suddenly losing my appetite. The science guy, whom I had hoped could give me orgasmic stem cells or something, is giving the same old recommendation: a vibrator.

"Because weak ones, you know . . . it should thump," he says. "It should give you a good thumping, not just a buzz but a thumping buzz."

He puts down his utensils, moves his plate aside so a square of bare table is uncovered. "It should go like this," he says as he pounds the empty space with his fist until our silverware rattles.

I look uncomfortably at our neighbors, worried they might catch on to our discussion. I quickly change the subject.

As we end our meal with dollops of complimentary mango ice cream, he tells me he'll get ahold of me as soon as funding comes through. He can't wait to get me into that fMRI machine to see what my brain-to-crotch connection is up to. And I can't wait to go home and hide under my bed. I feel a long, long way from coming, let alone coming in a machine.

WHERE'S THE KEY TO MY CLI-TAURUS?

BAGGAGE

I live in Brooklyn, on the top floor of an old brownstone. I have a panoramic view of lower Manhattan. The buildings jut into the sky; the sunset envelops the landscape; the last sunrays reflect off the windows and turn me, my legs dangling from the fire escape, a radioactive pink. I look out at all the lights flickering on and wonder how many women are orgasming in the city—out of eight million people, there are roughly four million vulva owners with the potential. I don't hear anything but cars zooming by, yet I am positive there is a lot of moaning going on. When I'm on the sidelines, I'm always more attuned to what others are doing.

Like Carl, whom I call The Collector. He lives in the basement and has an obsessive hoarding disorder; he keeps and collects everything. From my windowsill, I count the white, black, and plaid zipper bags he piles up on his patio. Once the heap reaches the second floor, a big semi truck comes and whisks it all away. Once it's gone, he starts again with one bag up against the corner wall.

It'd be nice if when his semi comes, it could also vacuum away some of the baggage pent up in my brain.

Each of the three girls who previously lived in my room moved out before a year was up to live with newfound fiancés. The room had magical man-finding power—well, until I moved in. To mark the anniversary of my move-in, I celebrated my ability to break magic-man-finding spells by buying a cheap Cabernet at the corner wine store, where I also like to go and check out the guys who work there. They are all nice, cute, and stylish. I think they are also all gay.

But I don't need a guy anyway. I'm busy.

Ever seen what happens to couples? First they fawn, then they fester, and then they fall apart. My best friend, Fiona, has been going through the various stages since we were six years old—her first relationship took place all in the course of a tetherball game. She recently got married after only two months of knowing Pedro. Her orgasms with him are the best she's ever had, she says, and his penis is huge. When she asked for my blessing, I told her, "You can always get divorced." She said it was the best blessing anyone had ever given her. I've had my share of relationships, but luckily she's had enough for both of us—those stages take up a lot of time and I only have one lifetime to get where I'm going. And I am trying to go somewhere.

Though I'm not actively seeking a boyfriend, I have to admit that I sleep with a stuffed elephant named Earl. I often wake up with his fuzzy trunk firmly gripped in my hand. I wonder if my subconscious is trying to tell me something.

I'd probably go gay too, if I were a guy. A simple and straight-forward hand job gets a penis off easy—I wouldn't have to contend with that confounding and complicated lump of squish you find between a female's legs. My legs.

Men are so uncomplicated that they have to unleash it in playgrounds, in parks, and on beaches for an added challenge. I remember when I was ten years old, at the La Jolla tide pools in California, a dude took out his cock and caressed it proudly in front of me, like a girl would touch her shiny ponytail. I was upset—and rightfully so. The penis was a monster, as long as my torso.

"I saw a stranger's penis!" I yelled to my parents.

They patted me on the back, trying to calm me.

I spent our dinner that night doodling lighthouses: tall, cylindrical bases with triangular roofs. My dad leaned over my phallic sketches and said, "Working it out subconsciously, huh?"

And maybe I'm still working out how uncomplicated men are; one of my recurring doodles is a palm tree flanked by coconuts.

I met my two roommates through Craigslist. They're in their early thirties. Leigh is a designer who's looking for a man. We talk about being fat, thinking we're fat, and getting rid of fat, usually while consuming something high in fat. My other roommate, Ursula, is a former investment banker turned documentary filmmaker. She has the three cats I mentioned before: Buddy, Sika, and Lucy. Pussies and I don't usually get along (in more ways than one), as was evident when one of them shat in my bed my first week of living here, but by unwilling association, I have become a cat lady. I officially spend more time with cats than I do with men.

Ursula is the real cat lady, but despite common lore, she has a boyfriend. She's trying to decide whether or not to move in with him. I use my parents, Ken and Deena, as a comparison. They have been married for thirty-four years now and sometimes they seem like the same person: Keena. They talk in we-form. If Ursula's ready to cut herself in half—turn into Urs- or -ula—I tell her, by all means, cohabitate.

Fiona's favorite way to orgasm is with the aforementioned rabbit vibrator. Leigh says she orgasms best with a fair amount of wine beforehand. Ursula says she can think herself off, just concentrate on her genitals to the point where she'll spontaneously orgasm right there in her chair.

I have to admit, I'm feeling quite curious and more than a little deficient right now.

Fiona—like my mother, and like everyone else—always tells me I have to explore myself first before having an orgasm with a partner. But I'd always hoped some man would hit a bull's-eye and save me the trouble of exploring myself while I could be out exploring the world. There are a lot of things to do out there.

Such as being a cocktail waitress, which is what I've decided to do at two different bars now—ACE Bar and Bleecker Bar—while I put my journalism career on hold for the sake of an orgasm. The bars are both like Chuck E. Cheese for adults: They have arcade games, pool, Skee-Ball, and darts, but the biggest game by far is seeking out a mate for the night. My shifts are like watching a Discovery Channel special on the mating practices of our species, which isn't so different from my last job. I worked as a staff writer at the *Village Voice* for a year. I found myself unquenchably drawn to sex-related topics—pornogami (pornographic origami), the intersection of Seaman and Cumming Street (Fiona lived a block away), and the love life of a learning-disabled man in his thirties—until I got fired. The reason: taste.

Ever followed a group of retarded people around? I'm kind of envious of them; they're perpetually in seventh grade. They can be lewd, crass, publicly scratch their crotches—letting out their inner animals—with no consequences. They seem so comfortable being human, acting exactly how they feel.

BAGGAGE

Which is what it seems people at the bar are often trying to accomplish with the alcohol they consume. They're more or less in a suspended state of retardation with a complete lack of inhibition. You'd think having brains would make you smarter, but all it does is make you better at suppressing who you are.

Which might be why I have a red wine compulsion—just a glass or two a night—to remind me, or in some cases to help me forget, who I'm *supposed* to be.

As the jukebox plays the latest hits, men chug poisonous concoctions to break down their common sense so they can act on their impulses. And the girls want to break down their common sense too, so they bat their eyelashes, signaling the senseless boys to buy them drinks. Everyone wants their senses broken; you can't be full of senses and go home with a stranger because this common sense of ours has been ingrained to "just say NO" to almost every opportunity.

So I'm good at exploring other people's sexuality—at the bar and in newspaper form—but I've done a rather doltish job of examining my own. I blame my common sense, among other things, for preventing my orgasm.

The radioactive pink of the sky turns more of a purple. I have these little fibers floating around in my eye's vitreous jelly. My cousin, who's an optometrist, told me most people have them—she calls them floaters—but learn to ignore them. For me, the cobweb-like strands projecting haphazardly upon my view are as apparent as a fluorescent road sign. They remind me that people, even if looking at the same world, will have different perspectives. Right now, as I scan the horizon, my floaters are misbehaving, getting all erratic like fireworks. I cross my fingers, hoping they are foreshadowing what will soon occur in my crotchular region.

CAPITAL LETTERS

I broached the idea with my family of writing about my search for orgasm. They all reacted a bit differently but mostly in ways that exhibited their openness with sexuality.

First of all, my parents were unsurprised about my orgasmic difficulties.

"We've always known you were a late bloomer," my mom said. My dad agreed. They almost always agree. They're Keena, remember.

The late-bloomer refrain is the most played-out phrase of my life. I was still getting head pats and my cheeks pinched at eighteen. Know what Fiona was doing then? Having orgasms.

I wasn't too worried about my parents' reactions; I figured they would be supportive. Sometimes I think it's *that* support that's at the root of my problem. Though their bellbottoms are moth-eaten by now, they're still free-love hippies at heart. They even dropped out of Berkeley together during the sixties.

There were signs my parents were different, but I could never really express it in words. When other kids' moms waved them down on the playground, there was a bare armpit. When my mom did the same, I saw that she had sprouted a toupee-type thing in the same location. I tried to teach her to wave with her elbow stuck against her ribs, while she tried to convince me that all women had hair under their arms and were supposed to leave it there. The scientific method made me question her conviction until I was eleven and I finally procured firm evidence: a babysitter shaving her pits in front of me.

My parents now have a plant nursery, but before that my father got his Ph.D. in psychology with an emphasis in sex therapy. I always bragged about my father's early occupation, thinking it was cool, but I never asked any details—the rumors were enough to fulfill my curiosity. I'd heard a story about my parents volunteering to be the models for a sex lecture series when they were younger. Slide after slide on a projection screen, they demonstrated the finer coital postures to undergraduate students. I never asked for the particulars, however, fearing they'd whip out the video and hold a screening party.

They told my two brothers and me everything about sex. In fact, I don't remember a time when I didn't know where babies come from. I was proud to know the facts of life when others my age couldn't even fathom them. Imagine the faces of all the other Brownies when I discussed the finer points of procreation around a campfire while we were supposed to be singing "Kumbaya." I rarely sang the song anyway. I had a hard enough time reciting the "under God" part in the Pledge of Allegiance every morning at school. In a largely conservative Christian area, I was raised as a cultural Jew and told that my one religious duty was to demand that my elementary school teachers supply me with blue and white clay—the Chanukah colors—instead of red and green, to make our customary Santa Claus tree ornaments. (It was my mom's way of showing my teachers that there was more than one way to be.) But back to the coital talks I gave to my fellow Girl Scouts.

"Your mom's wrong," I said. "The daddy sticks his thingy up her thingy."

I demonstrated with the s'mores skewer and the marshmallow. After that move, there was no more debate, just silence and a scowl on the troop leader's face.

If you really think about it—and I have—my parents now make their living off plant sex. Sometimes I think they chose the nursery profession because it's the only way they could legally engage in some sort of breeding all day long and still make money. After all, when we were growing up, our dinner table conversations consisted of vocabulary like propagation, fertilization, cross-pollination, hybridization, and germination (and much of the time it didn't even concern plants).

My theory is that Keena was too open about sex and I rebelled against it. It's like when you don't let kids have sugar cereals or watch TV and then all they do when they go to college is eat Fruity Pebbles and TiVo every show. Maybe my timidity about my own sexuality is actually a demonstration of the revolutionary within me.

Here's a contradiction of mine for you: though I'm timid in my own personal affairs, I can act with ease and comfort when dealing with others' sexuality. I feel almost as though talking so much about sex as a kid made it a logical, cerebral activity for me but left me unable to embrace its carnality.

So when I pitched the idea of a book to my parents, they got excited. In fact, my father started helping me with the research. He sent me all kinds of sex-related articles that he found in newspapers. The last one was from his local paper in San Diego, the *North County Times*, and it was about objectophilia, people who develop romantic relationships with objects. One woman was infatuated with a Hammond organ and feared infidelity when a technician performed repairs. He also sent me a catalog, which touted sex education films. Thanks, Dad.

My mom approached my project like it would yield the next Great American Novel, never mind that it's not a novel. She's extremely supportive and hopes that once I iron out my orgasmic wrinkle, grandkids will be on the way.

They only had one warning: Don't put orgasm in capital letters. Like this: ORGASM.

It's Keena's favorite expression: They're always telling me not to put things in capital letters. I think it's supposed to be a perspective-finder. It's their figurative way of saying, "Don't sweat the small stuff," and to them, everything is small stuff. My dad has bad eyesight, and when I put on his thick glasses, the world turns into one big, steep San Francisco hill. I wonder if this precipitous perspective has anything to do with his no-nonsense mentality. Worrying about things is unnecessary. Everyone should just get on with it already, slide down that inevitable hill of life and enjoy it, because at the bottom there's nothing to do but rot in the ground. Putting things in capital letters only causes bumps in what could otherwise be a smooth ride.

I don't always agree.

ORGASM—see?

I have my own perspective-finder anyway. It's the ant tattoo I got on my forearm. I look at it when I get anxious because it reminds me that at least I don't have to be worried about being fatally crushed by a shoe. But lately all it's done is make me wonder about ant sex. They're so tiny—how do they get it on?

My two older brothers had their own responses to my project, as well. Logan, who's just a year older, supportively said, "Go, sis, go get that O!"

But Matt, who's the oldest and also a natural-born specialist at provoking his younger siblings, taunted me. "Everyone's going to think you're a whore," he said. "No offense. I'm just getting you prepared."

UNREQUITED ORGASMS

Not only are my parents open about their sexuality, they're also in love to the point that it's kind of sickening. Keena met at Venice High School in Los Angeles and by my age already had their first baby.

They're inseparable. Keena works together; Keena sleeps together; Keena eats together. You'd think breakfast and dinner would be enough, but no, Keena even schedules lunch together at work. If my mom wants to take a shower, my dad tells her to wait up so Keena can take it together. I grew up believing married people weren't allowed to take showers apart. Seriously.

I recently was talking to my mother on the phone about relationships, and she prattled on about my father like he was a newfound infatuation. She gleefully told me about how he chases her up and down the stairs.

"You think I don't know that?" I said.

She paused, quizzically.

"Mom, I lived with you for seventeen years, remember?" I said. "The stairs are right by my old room. I could hear."

"Oops, you're right," she said, laughing spasmodically.

If they were really responsible parents, they would have set a more realistic example. Do they realize how high my romantic expectations are? What they have seems unattainable in this day and age. *Be normal! Get a divorce or cheat on each other. Come on, at least throw a plate at each other's head once in a while.*

One time I confronted them about their unattainable perfection.

"Don't put our relationship in capital letters," Keena said.

Growing up with that kind of example, I came to believe nothing could match it—even my friends said it was the most beautiful partnership they'd ever seen. I also thought love and orgasm were inextricably intertwined—orgasm came out of love; it wasn't something you did to yourself—and it seemed so clear that I never questioned the connection. So when I fell in love for the first time at seventeen, I was convinced my first orgasm would inevitably follow. Evan and I dated as seniors in high school and quickly gave each other the "first love" title. He was beautiful: olive skin that felt like crushed velvet, chiseled chin that we put a piercing in, a lanky cross-country-runner body that was perfect for me to lie on, and eyes that remained happy even when he frowned.

We carefully scheduled our first coital interaction, even discussed the background music: "Satellite" by Dave Matthews Band. I pressed play as he fiddled with the condom. The only witnesses were the glowing insect stickers I'd placed randomly all over my ceiling—and my lizard, a bearded dragon named Velcro, sitting silently in her aquarium.

The next day, I proudly told my mom what had happened. In response, my parents gave me their dog-eared copy of the Kama Sutra. Keena told me to enjoy sex, not to put it in capital letters; it didn't have to be a tremendous deal. But it was, because I was in LOVE.

In the ensuing months, I expected the O—that Big O people talked about—to show up. Because I somehow came to think of my coming as the guy's responsibility, I told Evan he was failing and would be in charge of purchasing all the condoms until I came. He orgasmed during sex, so why couldn't I? We were equals, right? All the many waves of feminism had told us that already. (After our breakup, when I wanted to be super-masochistic, I used to imagine Evan with a sassy lady who bought condoms in Costco value packs, made porn star noises, and arched her back like an ecstatic yogi in upward dog—that was her having multiple orgasms. His eyes and mouth smiled in unison when that occurred.)

Evan and I experimented and had fun. I always felt ecstasy in an emotional sense, but I kept wondering when the physical eruption would happen. The idea that virgins, locked in their bedrooms with nothing but their own fingers, could be having orgasms when I wasn't didn't even cross my mind. Orgasm with anything else but love seemed like an oxymoron.

My relationship, at the time, reminded me of my mother and father's. I became enamored of the idea that I'd found my mate and that we mirrored the ultimate model relationship in my life. Like my parents, we became one—Marvan or Evra. We lost our identities in our oneness and relished every moment of it. I dropped my friends in a second to be with him. I dropped my boundaries to build new ones around us both. I dropped my everything to be his everything. I thought that's how it was supposed to be.

We got into different colleges, me into UCLA and him to one up north, an eight-hour drive away. He compromised everything to come visit and even applied to transfer schools to be with me. When he got admitted, I severed the tie before he could pack up and move in. I was just too scared to share my identity so completely. I questioned how realistic it was for two beings to live and grow as one. It seemed like one part of the whole was often overwhelmed. Besides, there had to be more out there to do than to get married and plop out clones of me.

I don't know if it's symbolic or not, but I treat my relationships these days a lot like the plants my parents give me: I always forget to tend to them and they never last very long.

THE BLOSSOMED AND THE BUD

Fiona's been by my side through all my relationships—the last of which ended three months ago (but only lasted half of that). I haven't had a relationship for longer than two months since I was twenty-two (and that one lasted for three). Fiona thinks most of my relationships are self-sabotaged. Maybe they are, but I don't see how it was my fault that this last guy had an unappealing habit of eating an entire bag of Pepperidge Farm cookies in bed. Half the bag ended up in crumbs between my sheets. They poked at me, got stuck between my toes. Who'd blame me for putting a stop to that?

Fiona and I are pretty much always on the same page; our only problem is that we're often in different books. We met when we were six years old, and I was a bit of a runt. To help me reach the drinking fountain, she'd put me on her knee. If anyone else tried to pick me up, she'd deck them. When the gray-haired lunch lady pinched my cheeks and said she was going to take me home with her, Fiona would scowl and grab onto my arm to anchor me from being kidnapped. Twenty years later, she still looks out for my well-being.

We grew up two miles from each other on Buena Creek Road. She was raised Catholic and wasn't allowed to have a boy spend the night until she was out of her family's home, while my parents gave me the option to invite my first boyfriend to stay over before the thought had occurred to me. We both veered away from our parents' sexual norms. She was open and intuitively sexual, whereas I was timid. We had opposite color schemes too: She's a blue-eyed blonde with a porcelain glow. I'm olive-toned with wavy brown hair and eyes the color of an algae-infested pond when the sun shines through.

As early as second grade, our differences were becoming apparent. Fiona was already busy planning rendezvous with a fifth-grader named Mike, while I was in the cafeteria, fretting that I'd lost my plastic spork packaging. (I suffered from an overactive imagination, compounded by a fear of mortality, and worried that I may have inadvertently swallowed the plastic and forgot to choke.) While I employed the cafeteria staff to find my plastic wrapping, Fiona was having her first date.

That whole late-bloomer thing didn't help matters. Fiona, of course, sprouted into puberty like she was given Miracle-Gro. One time, we decided to compare how much pubic hair had grown in. We drew pictures. My little triangle was completely filled with pencil markings. When she turned hers around, there were only ten long spirals. At that point, I realized peach fuzz didn't count. I erased everything.

While I was more drawn to school, Fiona was beginning her acting and singing career. Her mom enrolled her in beauty pageants—she won Miss Pre-Teen San Diego and Miss Pre-Teen California. Instead of conforming to each other, we used our differences to define who we were. We created our identities off each other and stuck to our roles: she was the sexy one; I was the rambunctious one. For the past two decades, we've tried to coach each other: she constantly checks in to ensure my libido's pilot light remains lit, while I help her turn her flame down a notch.

Even to this day, she continues to stay ahead of me—see her recent marriage to Pedro. Really, the first thing she told me about him, which was a week before they got hitched, was about his crotchular gifts: his "dong makes her ding every time."

Fiona has tried to cure me, many times. She first got me a vibrator when we were seventeen and I'd first confessed my problem. It was in a purple case and it said Good and Plenty, but it yielded neither. I kept it in my underwear drawer for years and never even inserted a battery. It should still be there, in California, unless my parents have confiscated it or something. Fiona's given me other pointers. She told me about one of her favorite maneuvers: using the pressurized detachable faucet in her shower. I, however, have lived a life of exclusively anchored showerheads.

It would have been nice to know how to masturbate when, one time, I was in bed with a boyfriend and he asked me to masturbate in front of him. He said it turned him on. I wanted to please him but I declined, not knowing exactly how to go about it. Then I watched him jack off to Frank Sinatra with nothing but socks on.

It's not that I've never masturbated. I have masturbated. There—I said it. I've masturbated. Masturbation. Masturbate. I've masturbated, but it's always been half-assed. When I was younger, I'd use other objects for research, kind of like how my dog, Suzie, would use the back bumper of our Suburban to scratch her own back. I didn't run around town looking for phallic poles to sit on; I was subtler than that. As I rode my bike, I noticed that it felt good to put a little extra pressure against the seat as I turned left or right.

(I couldn't very well pull out a bike seat when my Sinatra-listening sock-clad boyfriend asked me to masturbate, could I?) I'd bunch up blankets and apply a pleasing amount of compression "down there," but I never went further than that.

Okay, I'm lying. I touched it once or twice, skin to skin, but I gave up. It grossed me out. *I* grossed me out. I was afraid of that part of my body and—let's face it—it's in a conveniently ignorable location. If I didn't explore down there, I never had to know if anything was wrong—or right—with it.

I wanted to employ Fiona to help me pick out that vibrator that Dr. Komisaruk became almost belligerent about, but unfortunately she's on an eight-month tour right now, flitting across the fifty states while playing the role of a snotty teenager onstage every night. She had to pack The Bullet and The Rabbit with an extra battery pack to keep her satisfied while separated from her husband's crotch.

A PORTRAIT OF AN ANORGASMIC

AS SEXUALLY UNSAVVY

I began playing obsessive-compulsive games with myself. *If I cross the street before the light turns red, I'll get my orgasm.* Then I'd sprint across to make sure I'd win. *If a red car passes me before I pass the third crack in the sidewalk, I won't get my orgasm.* No red car—I won again! Circumstances were looking pretty auspicious, except I wasn't making any tangible progress and I began questioning the state of my psychology. Can you be slightly OCD and not believe in a god? Because I was pretty sure stoplights and sidewalk aberrations had become my deities.

Knowing that my hang-ups were much more than physical, I decided to see a real therapist. I quickly and luckily found Rori. Her sofa chair dwarfed her. The blue cushioned arms came up to her shoulders. Her thick brown locks spiced up her appearance like a colorful throw rug would spice up a piece of furniture. The walls were all white except for one Van Gogh reproduction. I think it was supposed to be pacifying with its depiction of a flowing river, but the distinctive brush strokes reminded me of *The Scream*.

I snuggled into the side of the sofa and hugged a pillow tight. Then we stared at each other. She had no expression.

I bit at the side of my cheek, waiting for her to speak. I'm always gnawing or picking at something.

I started talking. I wanted to prove my damage, tell her as many things that were wrong with me as possible so she wouldn't think she was wasting her time. I told her about my orgasmic setbacks, my familial relationships, and different romances that had gone awry.

After a while, she went back to Evan, my first serious boyfriend. "What do you think about when you think of him?"

I clenched my teeth and thought for a while. My tongue discovered that my inner cheek lump had grown, in a short thirty-five minutes. I'd munched it into a welt the size of a single ball of salmon caviar.

"Don't think, just say what pops into your mind," she said.

"It was like I was a baby rattlesnake," I said. "I didn't know how much poison to let out, so I let it all out."

"You're talking about love as poison," said Rori. Then she spun my love metaphor back in my face. "What does poison do?"

"Kill," I said.

Damn, I'm a downer.

I told her my other first-love theory, hoping to appear more upbeat than a minute before, when I'd likened love to instantaneous death. I told her that first loves make a dent on the brain that can't be smoothed over. I smiled. *See that? That's better, right?*

"Are you listening to yourself?" she said. "A dent, like from a car accident?"

She had a point: All my talk was rather morbid for speaking about something as wholesome as love. But I was cynical about love these days. I explained the feeling I kept getting while serving drinks at the bar. I'd see all these happy couples everywhere and I'd think they were all just feeling love because it's an evolutionary tactic to ensnare us into procreating. We're just reproduction-bots. What if we could just send away for some seeds and smother them on terra-cotta and grow a child, hassle-free and emotion-free, like a Chia Pet? Then we could use all that angsty love energy to actually get somewhere.

Before I saw Rori, I'd wondered if I was really fucked up enough to see a therapist. By the time I left, I felt flawed enough to be a regular.

I exited the building. I went to cross the street. *If I jump three times and step on the curb with my right foot, everything will be okay. I'll get my orgasm.*

Talking about my past relationships brought up a lot of old memories. A part of me closed off after I lost my first love. I could've either been called a kissing whore or the queen of blue balls. I probably kissed more than half the college Ultimate Frisbee team, but I'd never do more than that. If I ever got into bed with a guy, I'd do cartwheels and somersaults right off the mattress—simultaneously enticing them with my acrobatic flexibility while making a getaway before any clothes were stripped off.

I went to Costa Rica during the summer of 2000; I was eighteen. There my mind expanded, but my labia majora stayed lip-locked. I dated Mario, a chestnut-brown resident of San Jose. His hair was long and wavy, each black strand as thick as four of mine. His eyebrows were like mink pelts. Mario would take a sip of lemon tea, and as a chaser, he'd have a snort of cocaine. That way he could have the stamina to play romantic songs with his garage band twenty-four hours a day. Drug users weren't as bad as the Disney after-school specials made them out to be, I found. And with coke that affordable down there, who could blame them?

About a month into our relationship, he made it clear he wanted to get more intimate. I told him I'd never had an orgasm before. This little fact always gets guys excited; it's like the twenty-first-century version of a virgin. He wanted to be my first—but it backfired. He told me the only way to achieve orgasm was not to use a condom. Shit! A cultural glitch. Safe-sex after-school specials had brainwashed me much better than the ones about drugs, and I refused. He was perplexed; his mink pelts closed in on each other, confounded. To him, safe sex meant pulling out; a condom represented mistrust. I wasn't about to head into my sophomore year at UCLA with herpes and a fetus. I'm sure they would have been great conversation pieces as far as souvenirs from Costa Rica go, but I stuck with bringing back coffee beans and a couple rolls of photos.

Brian was my next boyfriend. We started dating my sophomore year. He was four years older than I and was attending law school. I looked up to him more than I loved him. To him, I was probably something close to a cock-warmer. He knew all the right things to say, and everything about him was so straightforward. That was a warning: no human should make so much sense, and if he does, that means there's too much strategy. He didn't measure up to Evan, but I didn't have to worry about heartbreak anyway. I was leaving to go study abroad in Spain, so the relationship had a handy built-in expiration date.

He tried to get me off, but by this time I'd practically built an obstacle course around my clitoris. I got nervous with my own hands down there, much less anyone else's.

So we spent most of our time in the same old routine: missionary. Maybe he'd hit my G-spot, I thought. If man can land on the moon, is that too much to ask?

It was, apparently.

A PORTRAIT OF AN ANORGASMIC AS SEXUALLY UNSAVVY

I enjoyed being intimate with him, but when we got it on, I couldn't release my mind from the mundane. It was a self-fulfilling prophecy: I thought of myself as anorgasmic; therefore I was. I had moments when I watched the ceiling fan spin around as he was on top of me, talking dirty. I lay there trying to separate each blade by following it with my eyes like a cat would watch a windup toy. Other times, I felt that my anorgasmic sex was the result of not living in the moment, but I'd end up psyching myself out with my live-feed report: *Thrust.* No, no orgasm there. *Thrust.* Nope, still nothing. *Thrust.* Still no.

My cousin Nora gave me another option: faking it. "Just say, 'I'm coming, I'm coming,' then breathe heavy. Whip your head to the side, dig in your nails, and then play with your nipples until they're hard—you can't come without hard nipples. Contract your pussy. Then you're done."

"So, all you have to do is say that you're coming and they believe you?" I said.

"Pretty much, yeah," she said. "It's not very hard."

But I never built up the nerve to use her methods. Plus, what was the point? I wanted the real thing.

Other friends told me to get on top during sex. I never did because I don't have rhythm. I felt like he'd be looking up at me and I'd have to put on a theatrical, orgasmic performance—and I've never been much of an actress.

I pondered sex sounds. How does one make those? Is there a class I can take for that? And before I could ever come up with the answers, he'd already have rolled over and started snoring. *Wait, what'd I miss?*

I had a dry spell during my junior year abroad in Spain. Looking back at the photos, it appears I was rather focused on gaining weight, which I did very well. I attended classes there and had a concentration in beer and tapas. My Aunt Judy took pity on me for my lack of male contact, and that's how my second vibrator came into my life; she sent it first-class across the Atlantic. It was big, fluorescent, and purple. It had spiral rings around it and was appropriately called the Saturn. But even if I wanted to try it, I couldn't. It became a centerpiece on my mantle and a household favorite. While smoking joints, my roommates would pass it around and trip out as they clicked through its various speeds.

When I came home for my final year at UCLA, I missed penis. That's where my half, of the five and a half, comes in. You know the halves: the type that happen on days like your twenty-first birthday. Then you wake up the next morning with a thudding headache, smelling an old friend's halitosis. This person happens to be snoring on the pillow next to you, and after vague flashes of stuck zippers and tripping over your own underwear, you are almost positive something was penetrated. There's a half for you. Or my half for you, at least.

I graduated college with no job and no idea what to do. So I decided to fly off to India to find a job, which was the start of many travels around the world.

CAN'T OUTSOURCE ORGASM

If I had realized that street dogs' breeding activities were an indicator of sex in India, I would have known straight off that getting involved with anyone would be a complicated matter. Frequently, after one has humped another, the male's pink-tipped schlong gets stuck and the dogs wind up butt to butt, both trying to run in opposing directions. At most, they can muster an awkward sashay, and at the least, they bark and whimper. In India, they are all making babies, trying to keep up the species, but they look away from each other as if intercourse isn't actually what is happening.

Likewise, my time in India did nothing to enlighten my genitalia. There was no nirvana for my vulva. I think it made my pussy crawl even farther up inside me, if it's possible for a pussy to do that. When I arrived in Bangalore, I was twenty-one years old. I started working at an English daily newspaper, my first newspaper job. All the other staff members were Indian. We had many differences. For starters, they didn't see the importance of my first story: men who piss in the streets and the women who disdain them.

"It's not news," my editor said. "Men have been urinating in the street since the beginning of time."

Somehow, I got them to let me do the piece anyway.

Another difference became apparent within the gridlock at the back of the newspaper, filled with advertisements for wannabe wives and husbands. Arranged marriages were still commonplace, though growing less and less so in places with Western influence. I found it so odd, and so sad. What about love? You know, the kind that makes you forget yourself, do really dumb shit, and become blind to all your partner's faults? Isn't that what real love is about? All these people here, a whole country of them, were missing out, I felt. Although, on the other hand, there was a plus: I thought maybe they didn't have to worry about winding up jaded, like me.

But arranged marriages didn't stop sexual desire, as far as I could tell. There seemed to be so much repression that a lot of men didn't dare check out a woman in a sari, but when it came to the "loose Western girl"—me—they appraised my ripeness as conspicuously as they would a melon's, squeezing my ass a few times. Eyes were constantly aimed in my direction. When I would sit in the back of a rickshaw at a traffic light, all the men's motorcycle mirrors would shift, and instead of foreheads, chins, or ears, I'd suddenly see dozens of eyes reflected in my direction. I started to feel defensive. I expected that any man who talked to me only did so because he wanted something. My gender was a hindrance of a kind I'd never felt before.

Maybe a lot of the attention was my fault since I didn't know how to dress. I was wearing what I thought were big baggy things to the office, but my editor pulled me aside to tell me that my jeans and T-shirts were too alluring. I was going to have to get a more modest wardrobe if I wanted to continue working there.

CAN'T OUTSOURCE ORGASM

I had to be guarded because I didn't know how to interpret gestures anymore. I expected the worst from everyone. One time I went on a weekend journey by myself. I felt like going on a pilgrimage, so I looked in my guidebook for the nearest one: Thiruvannamalai, where people worship the Hindu god Shiva by circumambulating Arunachala Hill. On the way there, I had to stand on the bus. A saffron-robed sadhu, a holy man, stood behind me, and I swore he was trying to poke his "homo erectus" into me at every slight jolt. It caused a domino effect in which I instinctively shot my pelvis forward, making the person in front of me do the same, until it was like the wave at a baseball game. Some—me—would have said we looked like a bunch of nymphoma-niac dry-humpers on the way to their biggest festival of the year. But in reality, that sadhu was probably just trying to stay steady on his feet.

Soon after, while reporting a story about where to find the best masala dosa in town, I spied a man standing confidently near a tub of spiced potatoes. Amit wore a T-shirt, jeans, and Converse sneak-ers. I imagined that he was just like his wardrobe—very Western-ized. As we started chatting, I felt like I'd finally found someone who could, at least, understand me a bit. When he asked me out on a date, I was flattered. I didn't hesitate to say yes. I suspected that we had some fundamental beliefs in common—that a woman was lib-erated enough to walk alone on the street at night, for instance. The following week, we shared a great dinner—he'd had a friend open his restaurant late, just for us—and then we took a rickshaw back to his house to sit and talk. Once he got me there, he turned the bolt.

I'm not going to give you the details because they suck. He sucked. The raunchy asshole tried to . . . you know what he tried to do. But I yelled. I have lungs when I need to. I was lucky. I kicked, I screamed, but mostly I ran.

His thumbprint was imprinted on my forearm. A big blue dot. On the second day it turned greenish. It was yellowish and almost gone by day four, but unfortunately the experience wasn't. It stuck in my head, reminding me to challenge every assumption I made about new people and not to judge them by their T-shirts. But mostly I tried to hide my femininity, which seemed, at the time, the easiest way to stay out of trouble.

I closed up even more when I saw that it wasn't just me but other women who were also getting screwed—literally and figuratively—when they trusted men. In a small village in Tamil Nadu called Mahabalipuram, I went home with a woman who sold textiles on the street. She said if I paid for the ingredients, she would cook me a meal. She led me to a shack made of corrugated metal, its floor made of tightly packed dirt. We had to duck at all times since the ceiling wasn't high enough for us to stand up. As she rolled out bug-imbedded dough for our naan, she pointed to a photo on the wall. It depicted a tall white man with John Lennon–type glasses, disheveled hair, and a backpack. I thought I had finally figured out why she had brought me there. "Have you seen him?" she asked.

I narrowed my eyes and was going to laugh—how ridiculous to think I'd know some random dude on her wall just because he was white!—but then a toddler entered the room. Her skin was ten shades lighter than everyone else's—milk chocolate among pure cocoa. The textile vendor's daughter, who was about my age, followed the toddler inside and fixated on the photo. She started crying and begged me to buy her a beer. I didn't know if she'd been raped or paid or promised a new life in a richer country. Maybe her circumstances were the same as mine were with Amit but she was just less lucky. I bought her a liter of Kingfisher. She downed it in a few gulps and quickly asked for another.

"He's the bad man," said the older woman. "If you see him, tell him he has a daughter in Mahabalipuram. We wait every day for him to return." And with that, she nodded her head in a way that was at once defeated and defiant.

And so, after this harsh education in sexual relations, it was very odd and unexpected when I met Rafiq, a thirty-year-old Muslim man with an eighties-style bushy mustache he liked to call his "mouche." Every time I saw him, my eyes went dry (I'll let you guess where the moisture went). I never expected to be attracted to someone like him. He was the opposite of just about everyone who'd ever turned me on—more naïve and innocent than even I was. He was a backcountry guy who had come to the city to support his family. He had eight siblings, all in a town a three-hour bus journey away. On a $150 monthly salary, he was desperately trying to save enough money to pay his sisters' dowries. Rafiq swore they'd all be married off before he got a wife for himself.

Rafiq and I worked at the same paper. He was about half my thickness—I could wrap my thumb and forefinger around his wrist. He'd rather save a couple extra rupees for his family than sit down and eat. He had only two shirts and two pairs of pants, but he came to work each day looking as though each garment had been dry-cleaned and hand-pressed. He'd sit at his computer, typing out a story with deliberate pokes, as if his fingers were bird beaks feeding on a pile of lettered seed. His glasses were always a bit crooked, and because he was a foot taller than I was, I could never figure out if it was his ears or the spectacles themselves that were lopsided. "Your glasses are crooked"—that's how I broke the ice, one morning.

We started with small chitchats during lunch. He'd smoke a cigarette while I sipped down my milky tea. His heavy accent could be hard to follow—he spoke primarily in Urdu and Kannada—but I enjoyed listening anyway. I could sway to his singsong lilt and nod encouragingly. We went on an assignment together. It was the typical story done each year after Diwali, the festival where people, especially children, light up fireworks in the street. We went to various emergency rooms around the city to count how many eyes had been blown out. Despite the dozen or so kids we saw with bandages around their heads, we had a truly great night. He seemed to want only to know me, nothing more. I liked that.

It was soon Ramadan, and Rafiq was heading home to visit his family. He asked if I would like to see his hometown. At the time I had no idea what that meant. On our way there, Rafiq told me that his father was an imam. Being aware of the Palestinian-Israeli conflict, but not much else about Muslim-Jewish relations, I thought his father was going to shoot me as soon as I reached his foyer.

We arrived while it was still night out. Rafiq's mother and sisters practiced purdah, meaning they wore burkas when outside and stayed hidden when male strangers came into the home. They spoke little English but conveyed soon enough that they wanted to check out my legs. They laughed, smiled, pointed, and pretty much squinted at the white glare emanating from my calves. They asked which caste I was from, which could translate to "Which religion do you practice?" I looked over at Rafiq's father, who was sitting in a chair. I was glad he was sitting down for this. His stark-white *kurta* matched his beard. His eyes stared straight toward me, but he couldn't see; they were fogged over with cataracts. Only his pupils were visible, like stray birds passing fluffy clouds. As I told them I was Jewish, I cringed, expecting the worst, but they just bobbed their heads back and forth, laughed, and then motioned for me to roll up my pant cuffs again.

It was almost dawn, so we hurried to eat *sahari*, the breakfast served before a long day of fasting. Rafiq's mother was the type who wouldn't take no for an answer. "Eat more, eat more!" she exclaimed. She served me about a pound of rice, four types of chutney, and a bowl of *baingan bharta* (roasted eggplant with spices) and watched me eat until the top button on my jeans was about to pop off. (An hour or so later, I was inclined to nickname her dish baingan farta. I was the only one who thought that was funny. Everyone else burped.)

It took about forty-five seconds to show me around the house. There was one shared room, and we had just eaten on its floor. The kitchen area had a little shower curtain pinned up for separation, and the tiny closet had a hole and a bucket where, apparently, they all went to the bathroom. They asked if I wanted to wash up. "No, I'm fine." I didn't want to figure out how to scrub in a place so confined.

After a long day of checking out the town, Rafiq and I returned to his home for dinner. I was starving. We broke fast with a voluptuous date and warm, sweetened milk. Then we ate *iftar*. There were so many plates of food on the ground that there was hardly enough room for all twelve of us to sit. After dinner, his sisters dressed me in a burka. They fussed around with how it lay on my hips, made me spin around, and then told me I was "the most beautiful." I didn't know how to take that exactly—I was one big black blob. Even my eyes were covered. (Later I found out that Rafiq's favorite outfit of mine was a huge shapeless yellow raincoat I wore during monsoon season. The more I had on, the more turned on he'd get, apparently.) As I peeled off the burka, they asked me one more time, "You want to wash up?"

"No, I'm fine. Thank you very much."

Everyone got ready for bed. That meant rolling up the mat where we had just eaten dinner and substituting another mat where everyone would sleep crammed together like crayons in a box. Meanwhile, Rafiq and I climbed up to the roof. We looked at the neighboring buildings as the call to prayer began. Men slipped out of all the adjacent houses and paraded toward the mosque, with its minaret jutting upward, for the last prayer of the day. As they did, Rafiq stayed near me. It was too romantic. I kissed him. He pointed to his heart.

"You are right here now," he said. "The world looks different. I love you, you are my Mara."

"No, you don't *love* me," I said. "You *like* me."

I refused to use the word "love." It was just too serious for me. I knew from experience where that led.

His mother climbed up to check on us. I wanted to bang my head against the ground. It was true: American girls *are* a bad influence. We're loose.

When she left, Rafiq told me he'd let me know when it was time to be married. I started choking on my saliva as we climbed back down the stairs to go to bed.

The next morning, Rafiq had to do some errands around town. I stayed home with his sisters and mother. When I looked outside, I saw his youngest brother riding around on a camel in the front yard. They asked me if I wanted the next ride. "Maybe next time," I said.

We prepared the food for the evening. I began crying. I was confused and unsure why the tears were coming. Was it hunger, the idea that I might have unintentionally become a fiancée, or just the juicy onion on my cutting board? Rafiq's mother told me not to cry. "I love you more than my own daughters," she said. I looked at her daughters. They looked at me. Then I started to cry even harder. Where was I? What was I doing?

Before Rafiq came home, she asked me one more time if I wanted to wash. I noticed they all had the same clothes on as when I first arrived. "Why should I wash if you all aren't washing?" I asked.

"When we have guests," she said, "we do as they do."

Oy vey!

CAN'T OUTSOURCE ORGASM

Rafiq finally came home and we had another filling dinner before hopping back on the bus to Bangalore. On the way home, we held hands, but I couldn't help but think I'd done something wrong. He told me that I was his first kiss.

"*First?*"

"A kiss means very much, nah?" he asked. "Doesn't it?"

I realized kissing was in capital letters to him. Like this: KISS.

I'd never really thought so deeply about what a kiss meant. If I had, I wouldn't have had time to kiss all the men in my past.

When we got back to Bangalore, I had some housing issues. I ended up staying with Rafiq in his little hovel just outside the city. The walls were turquoise with pink trim. He had no furniture, only newspaper scattered here and there and a clothesline strung from door to window. The only decorations were two See's Candies boxes stapled to the wall, which my brother had brought when he visited from California, with "Sweet Memories" inscribed by Rafiq in permanent marker across the top. We slept on the tile, just a thin blanket beneath us. It was so hard I got bruises on my hips from tossing and turning. The bathroom was outside, and we took showers with a bucket. He'd heat my water with a plug-in warming wand, but he'd take his bucket-washings cold, like a man. Our pastime was kicking cockroaches into the corners.

No one from work knew about our arrangement. It would have been considered extremely inappropriate. We carried on the way we had before, a milky tea and cigarette lunch break. The only touching I saw in public occurred between members of the same sex. The men would hold hands, hug, and even stand one in back of the other. It didn't mean they were gay; it was just a way to deal with feeling deprived of intimate contact. But the staring continued. There were times when I longed for that burka again. I started thinking of it as a thin black force field. When Rafiq and I got home, we'd make up for lost time and indulge in our intimacy, which was about the only thing we had. I learned the critical age to acquire kissing skills is much beyond that for language; he caught on quickly. For a long time our physicality never strayed beyond caresses and kisses. He liked it when I'd say "Allah" and then rub his shoulders; he'd laugh, his "mouche" teetering precariously.

Rafiq said he didn't know what sex was until he was in his late teens; from behind the kitchen curtain, he overheard his mother giving his oldest sister her wedding night instructions. He was taught never to touch himself. He said masturbation was against his religion. I asked him if he ever did it anyway. He said he didn't want to think of touching "it" (finally, we really did have something in common). When I said maybe he should just give it a whirl, he asked if it would hurt. I thought he could use a lesson. I whipped out a condom, snuggled crisply in my backpack. I opened it and demonstrated, on my finger, the right way to use prophylactics. He got grossed out at the spermicidal lubricant and hopped to the other side of the room. So here I was, a bit of a prude myself, to say the least, meeting a man less sexually realized than myself. And I'd become the teacher.

But what I had hoped to achieve for years, he achieved in seconds. Except he couldn't even appreciate the feeling. "I felt like I had to pee," he said, laughing with embarrassment and bobbing his head after his first hand job. So that wasn't exactly a turn-on.

While his lack of experience was a problem for me, my experience was a problem for him. I wrote a story looking into how reliable HIV clinics were and if they adhered to protocol. I got Rafiq to be my accomplice; he went in and got tested, pretending he'd been with whores in Mumbai. After the test, we had our cigarette and tea. He implied that I, of course, didn't need the test because I'd never had sex before either. I said, "Well, actually . . ." He couldn't speak to me for about two days. It wasn't out of anger, but rather complete shock and horror at how I could have been a coconspirator in losing my own dignity.

He soon recovered, but the closer he got to me, the more I felt myself moving away. His sweetness was suffocating. His eagerness became off-putting. The oneness was threatening. He'd call me his sweet ladoo, after an Indian dessert made of ghee, flour, sugar, and other things all mushed together into a tight little ball. He'd constantly say, "I love you," and I'd return the compliment with, "Don't say that please." We had fun together, but it became increasingly frustrating; it would sometimes take twenty minutes to communicate a simple sentence. Quite often, instead of saying what I wanted, I would remain silent so I didn't have to put in the effort to explain. When I got frustrated, he seemed to like me more for it. "People only yell at the people they love most, don't they?" he'd say. I didn't like who I'd become. We were like the street dogs: side by side temporarily, brought together by circumstance, but inevitably bound to go different ways.

As I was leaving a few months later, he bolted through the security barricade in front of my gate and waved me down. He wanted to direct one more "I love you" toward me. "Oh, Allah," I said exasperatedly, "don't say that please." I turned away.

I had plans to go back to work in India after spending a month at home and renewing my work visa. But as I walked away, I felt so free that I wasn't sure I'd be able to return. I wanted Rafiq to get married, maybe the way it was supposed to be. All of a sudden arranged marriages started to make much more sense to me. There seemed to be no hurt or confusion, and maybe it was a way of staying safe from the illusions—or the unrealistic expectations—about what love could be.

Despite how close we got, Rafiq never touched me below the waist; I never let him. I kept telling myself I was doing him a favor by stopping his hands at my hips. If he didn't know what a kiss meant, then how would he interpret a crotch? It was the one thing, within the teeming throngs of difference and unfamiliarity, that I felt I could keep to myself.

FAIRY GODMOTHER OF MASTURBATION

Dr. Komisaruk had made the orgasm sound as simple as fishing—I get a hefty vibrator, cast it into my crotch, hook an orgasm, and reel it in—so I wanted to employ someone to help me pick out this thumping vibrator he was so adamant about. Fiona was still gone, in Chicago by now, so who better to help me than the Mother of Masturbation herself, Betty Dodson?

Betty Dodson is to masturbation what Mahatma Gandhi is to peaceful resistance, what Jennifer Aniston is to the shag haircut, what Pee-wee Herman is to indecent exposure—the words are virtually synonymous. You say the word "dildo" to anyone even tangentially related to the sex industry, and you get the same response: "Have you talked to Betty Dodson yet?" So I gave her a call.

It took awhile to whittle some time out of her. She was busy compiling an opus on orgasm information, but she finally agreed, in the name of sisterhood, to help me select my first vibrator.

Before making my pilgrimage to the great guru of clit, I read her book, *Sex for One*, which tells her masturbatory life story. Betty grew up in Kansas during the thirties and moved to New York in her twenties to become an artist. She thought a penis would give her an orgasm, just like I did, so she found one and married it. (Thankfully, I didn't go that far.) The orgasm of the day was vaginal; clitoral orgasm, according to Freud, was an immature way for a grown woman to come. But the penis didn't have Betty coming, and by the time she divorced, sexually dissatisfied, she was thirty-five. It was the sixties and the feminist movement was about to kick into high gear. Betty got involved and went gay for quite a number of years.

In 1973 she started BodySex workshops in her apartment. Women would gather and she'd teach them about their anatomy and how to masturbate with Hitachi Magic Wands. They all spread 'em for each other, checking one another out and snapping photos. They looked into their vulvas with mirrors. Betty described her labia as looking like the wattle on a chicken. They discovered that every vulva was unique, like a milk spill. They saw figs, flowers, orchids, and shells. Betty categorized some of the types: the Classical Cunt, with symmetry; a Baroque style with complex folds; a Gothic Cunt with archways; and a Danish Modern with clean lines. That was all very cute and good, but when I wondered what mine would look like, I was pretty sure it'd be something odd, outlandish, and outré like an Antoni Gaudí construction.

After years of leading the workshops, she retired and began private sessions. She now calls herself an "orgasm coach" and teaches self-love techniques for $1,100 per session, which can often span an entire afternoon. She's the CEO of masturbation.

I've needed a masturbation instructor for a while; the subject was never even addressed in sex-ed class. The only thing we learned in school about sex (besides recess conversations about who was doing what to whom in the spin-the-bottle sessions I wasn't yet developed

FAIRY GODMOTHER OF MASTURBATION

enough to be invited to) was how to take care of five-pound sacks of flour that our junior high sex-ed teacher, who was actually the science teacher, called "flour babies." It was no wonder my school had such a high rate of teenage pregnancy—everyone thought if they got sick of their baby they could mix it with eggs and milk and make muffins out of it.

I don't blame it on my teacher, though. She had to stick to the rules: we had an abstinence-only program, which didn't leave a lot of room for the clitoris.

I anxiously fumbled with my notepad as I stood in front of Betty's door. Maybe I wasn't yet ready for her, such a heavy hitter in the female orgasm field, so early on in my journey. I tried to prepare myself for anything: vibrators jumping around on the floor, hanging phallus mobiles ejaculating colorful laser lights, nude women lying on beanbags eating Cheetos and diagramming each other's vulvas with the remnant cheese powder on their hands.

I knocked. No one answered. I rang the doorbell. No one answered.

As I was turning around to go, the door opened.

I'd prepared myself for a lot of different scenarios, but not this one: A young man stood in the foyer in his butt-hugger black undies and a black T-shirt, through which shapely pectorals bulged. He was lanky and tall with curly brown hair and wire-rim glasses. The glasses sat atop a very beaky proboscis.

"Betty Dodson?" I said.

"Oh, you're here for the interview," he said. "I'm Eric, her assistant." He held out his hand for a shake. I received it, reluctantly. Can you trust a man when all he's got on are his underpants?

That was all I heard for a while. He said other stuff, but I wasn't paying attention; I was too busy staring at his package and wondering if I was going to be asked to strip down. What underwear did I have on? Shit, I hadn't coordinated. He pointed to the floor where there were a bunch of shoes lined up, so I slipped off my own. He led me to the living room. I stood in a daze. I took in only tiny fragments. There was blue carpet and plastic chairs against a wall. There was an ergonomic keyboard that Eric's hands sat poised on. A nude sketch of a woman on her side hung near a window. Lots of cunt jewelry: a jade cunt in a terra-cotta bowl, a silver cunt, cunt beads. Shelves lined with lubricants and oils. Stacked boxes of Hitachi Magic Wand massagers. A row of blown-glass phalluses on her mantel caught my attention. They each had an identical twin reflected in the mirror behind them. My eyes scanned up and down every one. Some were long and smooth with bulbous structures on the end. The one that most intrigued me had textured dots, almost like spines, running along its trunk and its translucent nut-sack—a cock cactus. My parents would have been pleased.

"You know what Betty likes to say about those," said Eric, checking me out as I checked them out.

"No," I said.

"That she's fucked all of them," he said, laughing. "It's great, she's got a story for each one. Who's fucked it. When they fucked it. Where they fucked it."

This wasn't exactly my type of humor, but I tried to laugh along as I stepped slowly away from him.

I never thought a big red velvet twat would be something that could relax me, but it did. I spotted a Wondrous Vulva Puppet, like the one I had bought from Dorrie Lane, on Betty's shelf. I started to stabilize, quite possibly drawing on my latent vulvalutionary power. Then a petite but sturdy woman with gray hair clipped short, calf-length stretch pants, a black shirt, and a phone to her ear popped out from the back room and waved me in.

FAIRY GODMOTHER OF MASTURBATION

Betty sat, and I found my own spot across from her. We were in her bedroom. There was only a computer, a desk, a big purple bed, and a Pilates ball in the corner. Betty is no longer the Mother of Masturbation—she's the Grandmother—but at seventy-eight years old, she looks not a day over sixty. Fondling the vulva might just be the antidote to aging. I wanted my orgasm now more than ever.

She dove right in. "So, you want to have an orgasm," she said. "See, I started masturbating when I was five. I've got my hand on my pussy, on my clitty, and I'm going, 'Oooh, it feels good,' and I call it my tickle, and my mom's like, 'Yeah, it feels good, doesn't it?' That's the natural way we should grow up, but very few of us have had that opportunity."

"Actually, my parents were very open," I said.

"Oh, you're one of those," she said. "You had to be opposite. They hate sex, you love sex. They love sex, you hate sex. How old are you?"

"Twenty-six."

"Late bloomer," she said.

I tried to bring us back to a little small talk, some level to relate on first. "I've got a vulva puppet too," I said, pointing to hers down the hall. "Mine's called Picchu."

"Oh yeah, from Dorrie," she said, of the puppet's innovator. "They're anatomically fucked up."

Betty rolled her chair toward her computer. She put on her glasses; they were shaped like a bra's underwire, two half circles cradling her eyes. She started scrolling through her Web page, acting very serious, like Dr. Masturbation. I had a vision of her holding a stethoscope to my clitoris, listening for a pulse.

I started to open up to her and told her all the things I wanted to do. I wanted to write about women and femininity and sexuality. I thought she'd understand, even cheer me on.

But she didn't. She was pushy, strong, and unyielding. She told me not to write a damn word yet.

"Get your orgasm first!" she demanded. "Orgasm is your grounding. It's your base to everything else."

She made it sound as if I were a lesser being because I'd never come. I think she noticed the look of despair on my face.

"Okay, just think of someone who hasn't had an orgasm," she said. She began channeling someone who hadn't orgasmed before. She pranced around in circles with limp wrists and talked in a baby voice.

"My sexuality is unknown to me," she cried. "I have no idea what it is and everywhere I look is sex sex sex. I'm innocent. I'm a victim. I'm dumb. I'm uninformed. I'm out of touch."

She sat back down.

"Could it be more obvious?"

I was having a hard time seeing her point. I had gone there for a vibrator, not to be torn apart.

"At twenty-six," she said, "you're coming off like fifteen or sixteen, like a teenager."

"Right now?" I said. "Sixteen?"

"You send off childlike vibes," she said. "You're very childlike. You start getting your orgasm going, you'll be a woman. But come on, you're a little baby girl now."

I think she was trying to taunt me into pulling down my pants right there and grabbing her dildos. It'd be another story for her collection. But no, I kept cool. Her honesty pleased me, but I had to admit, I was feeling defensive.

"I know stuff," I countered.

"You're smart," she said. "But you're not smart enough to know how to give yourself an orgasm." She laughed. She laughed for a long time.

FAIRY GODMOTHER OF MASTURBATION

She told me that as soon as I had my first orgasm, my energy would shift. "Your mommy and daddy are going to be very proud of you," she said. "You'll call them and say, 'Mother, Daddy, I'm ORGASMIC! I'm fucking everyone I can get my hands on in New York City!' Get it?"

Uh-huh.

I guess belittling you is just how she warms up, though, because afterward she began to act like the masturbatory role model I was hoping for—my fairy godmother of masturbation. She asked if I had a boyfriend. I said no. She said that was perfect because I needed to learn to love myself first, before I could tell my lover how to please me. (I'd heard that before, of course, but this time I planned to be more open to the advice.) She said so many girls these days think they'll fall in love and it will just happen; all they'll need is a penis and their vulvas will orgasm if it's Mr. Right. "None of that is true," she said. "The truth is that you'll get fucked and you won't come."

I tried to take the focus off me for a second. I asked her if our culture glorified one-night stands. I thought so. Every time I watched *Sex and the City*, I was envious that these women could hop into bed with a man of their choosing, get what they wanted out of it, and keep on moving. Her answer surprised me.

"I wish it did glorify one-night stands," she said. "But even Samantha would get drunk and look for Mr. Right. That's hardly the image of a liberated woman. That's a desperate woman. And in her real life, she's very monogamous and very married and very, very proper."

"Didn't she write a book about sex?"

"Yeah, and that's how unfucked this culture is," said Betty. "We take an actor who plays the role of a woman who has a lot of sex and now she's an expert."

I rolled that word around in my mouth for a while: unfucked unfucked unfucked.

That's what I felt like.

We settled back in front of her computer and started trouble-shooting the best way to get me "grounded." She said first off, it's very important to do Kegel exercises, the squeezing of the pubococcygeus muscles, which so many yoga teachers call the pelvic floor. She said they were the same muscles used to stop pee midstream. If I contracted and relaxed them over and over again, it would reduce my chances of urinary incontinence and up my sexual gratification ante.

"No one will even know you're doing it," she said. "You can do it on the subway or even in line at the grocery store."

She quickly moved on to more technical masturbatory issues; she said that after more than four decades of mulling masturbation over, she's decided that it's best to start off masturbating manually and steadily work your way up to increasingly more intense vibrators.

"Once you get used to something," she said, "it's hard to go back." She scrolled to a small device, a tad bit bigger than a nostril-hair trimmer.

"So here's the Water Dancer," she said. "A lot of women are in love with this."

She recommended the Dancer as a beginning vibrator, but she scrolled down and explained other models. We saw the Passionette, which has three speeds and is totally silent—good for a house with roommates. Next, the three-speed Strawberry appeared on the screen—it looked like a bike handle. Then we came upon a gigantic black rubber dildo, the Nimbus.

"This is the great big mother here that scares everyone," she said, laughing. The Nimbus, even in two-dimensional form, made me put my newly learned Kegels into practice; I clamped my pubo-coccygeus muscles so tightly shut that not even a slim-fit tampon would fit through. I relaxed a little when we came across a delicate yellow device.

"That thing doesn't do anything for me," Betty said. "But I'm an old warhorse."

When there were no more left, she gave me my last option. She brought her hand to her mouth. "You can also just spit on your hand and get your paw down there."

Betty said dildos come later but gave me some advice in the meantime. She recommended going to the grocery store and buying a bunch of phallic-shaped veggies: it's better to see what size fits best before investing in something more permanent. She said zucchinis are the most reliable vegetable but had one warning from her prior experiences: women's eyes are usually much bigger than their vaginas.

I asked her if there was a difference in the kind of orgasm I could have depending on the device I used.

"Honey," she said, "an orgasm is an orgasm is an orgasm. All that stuff about bigger and better and massive and the Big O—oh, come on, that's America. Just get an orgasm!"

She climbed on top of her desk. She began pulling DVDs from her shelf, ones she had made. She piled four into my arms—*Self-loving*, a video of a BodySex workshop; *Celebrating Orgasm*, showing her private sessions; *Orgasmic Women*, demonstrating thirteen different women's masturbating styles; and *Viva La Vulva*, a genital show and tell.

When she hopped back into her chair, she closed down her computer and looked at me. "Name your pussy, too," she advised. "Mine's Clitty Anne. My real name's Betty Anne, so: Clitty Anne."

"I'm Mara Rose," I said.

"Clitty Rose," she said. "That's good. Clitty Rose, I like it!"

We got up and she gave me a light spank. "Clitty Rose."

I was giddy. The Mother of Masturbation had just named my pussy. I felt like she'd anointed me as a disciple.

I asked her if she had sex anymore and if there were any tips she had. She said her life is sex, her work is sex, and usually that's enough to satisfy her, but when it's not, she's got Eric. "I live with this beautiful young man," she said, "and he's available whenever I want it."

I couldn't believe it. My circuits were too overwhelmed to open my mouth.

She spanked me again, nudging me toward the front living room. Our time was up. I spotted the dildos on her mantel again and just as I did, she started her story.

"You hear the joke I like to tell?" she asked, not hesitating long enough for me to tell her I had. "I've had sex with every one of those right there."

I didn't know what to say, so I asked her if she washed them afterward. As soon as the question left my lips I felt more like a sixteen-year-old than ever.

"No. I leave all the pussy juice on them so you can sniff it," she said, and like a bitchy older sister, she pushed me toward them. "Go over there and sniff 'em!" She laughed, hard.

It was tough love, but I knew she was on my side. She walked me toward the door and then assigned me homework. I had to watch the DVDs and get a mirror to investigate my body and all the parts that made up Clitty Rose.

"Get to know her," she said.

She said the only wrong way to masturbate was to get frustrated while masturbating—it takes time.

FAIRY GODMOTHER OF MASTURBATION

"Don't make it a chore. Just do it as often as you can," she said. "I don't do anything every day except for shit, eat, and sleep."

She said if her advice didn't work, she'd offer her services—and Eric's, too, as a surrogate sex partner. That frightened me more than the Nimbus, probably because Eric was sitting right next to me, smiling.

As I shuffled out the door, she called after me. "Make me proud!" she said. "Remember, if you want something done right, do it yourself!"

WIRED, UNWIRED,

AND THEN REWIRED AGAIN

When I got home from India, I couldn't go back. I didn't know how I would face Rafiq. He had become a distraction. Every day I'd stress about the story I was working on, or stress about figuring out my next one, and he tried to calm me. "You are going up too steep a hill," he'd say, moving his bony fingers vertically. "Go steady, you last longer that way." But I didn't want steady, I wanted to go higher, faster, farther. I couldn't go back, I'd been there before. I had to go forward. I had to progress.

I had applied to get my master's in journalism at Columbia University, and while I waited for the response to my application, I changed my return ticket from India so that it was Peru-bound. The roommates I'd had in Spain, the ones who loved the Saturn vibrator, had told me that Cuzco was the most magical place on Earth. I needed some magic to aid in my ambitions. I planned to become a hermit in a mountain-based hut and write my first novel. I didn't want any distractions, any romantic afflictions. I started the first few pages before I left. It was going to be about a girl who had to leave love in order to expand her horizons.

My friends, especially Fiona, told me that I was running away from something. That running-away talk, I said, was just a movie cliché. I wasn't running away from anything. I was finding something. What I was doing was called living.

In early 2004, at twenty-two years old, I landed in Cuzco, a small Andean town with more than three thousand years of history. It serves as a base for travelers on their way to Machu Picchu. It sits in the mountains, 10,912 feet above sea level. To keep my brain from feeling like it was going to leak out of my ears, I drank cup after cup of coca tea, which is made from the same plants as cocaine. The tea helps with altitude sickness. The indigenous people chew on the coca leaves almost religiously. For the already acclimated, the leaves stave off hunger and act as a coffeelike stimulant. After a while, they spit them out in what look like miniature piles of manure. I rented a little house on the side of a mountain. I counted once: there were about two hundred stairs and a steep incline to make it from the main plaza to my door. My ass got so tight that my cheeks defied gravity and were slowly working their way up my spine.

I began writing six to ten hours a day, hardly taking a look around. I only excused myself to go outside for provisions. After about three weeks of this routine, I ran into a pack of young Argentinean guys who'd been living in town for a few months. My Spanish was passable, so I chatted with them a bit.

Paco, Carlos, and George had moved to Cuzco for a new chance in the world. Back in Argentina they were having a hard time finding jobs. The country had had an economic crisis only a few years before, and the question plaguing many young adults was not what they *wanted* to be when they grew up, but what was in the classifieds.

Over the next week, they stopped by my house constantly. They roused me from my writing chair and made fun of me for working while the sun shined. They asked me what the point of working was if I wasn't going to have any fun. I said work was fun. They said what they heard of Americans must be true, then: *Americans live to work.*

They invited me to participate in their world for a day. They acted as my personal guides. We sat in a circle and they showed me how to drink yerba maté, a loose-leaf tea, which is drunk out of the cavernous bowl of a dried-out gourd. The gourds were as much a part of their bodies as any other extremity, attached at all times. It was a social ritual, but also a nice stimulant. We sat and talked for hours while Paco poured water, replenishing it as it was passed around to each person—each of us sipping out of the same metal straw. They told me about *breecheros,* the locals who hung out at the bars in hopes of going home with a foreigner for the night. The ultimate goal was to get a ticket out of the country; a close second was running away with a wallet full of cash. They took me to some temple ruins behind my house with nothing but the light of the stars and the sound of a flute to guide us. While Carlos brushed his hand lightly across my own, we made offerings of feathers and fresh flower petals to the Incan gods and goddesses.

I tried to get back to work, but day after day I found myself more tempted to go out and find them. When we explored the marketplace, I cursed my ass; it seemed to want to walk ahead of the boys and catch their attention. My hands were evil too; they kept frolicking in my hair, tossing it over my shoulder and tucking it behind my ears coquettishly. All my body parts were trying to sabotage me.

Then one day we all went up to a mountaintop with a shaman. It was raining lightly. And we staked out a spot with a tent and then proceeded to drink a boiled-down concoction made with a hallucinogenic cactus called San Pedro. Supposedly, we weren't doing it for the trip but for the enlightenment. Andeans use it traditionally to reach a spiritual healing state. The batch didn't work, but I was enlightened when Carlos started playing footsie with me in the tent.

I didn't get back to writing after that; my main character was left untransformed, an un-self-realized loveless chick, because Carlos had diverted my energies. What could I do? I became busy translating his eyelashes: they were so long that when he blinked in a certain manner, they communicated as much as his hands, which flailed around like an Italian in mid-speech. After the weight of India, Carlos lightened my load. Instead of being the bride-to-be, I'd watch him get stoned and cook large vats of stew for anyone brave enough to try whatever he'd concocted.

Carlos and I moved fast. He didn't seem to know more than two moves: kissing and intercourse.

You know when you're talking to someone in all sorts of boring platitudes and then you overhear tidbits of a really hot conversation right next to you, and you want to turn around and listen but you can't because it'd be rude? That's what sex had become for me. It's like I was stuck in a discussion with my internal monologue, which was full of boring, mundane crap, but couldn't help being distracted by snippets of the hot conversation going on down in my crotch. I couldn't figure out how to interrupt myself and become fully part of the discussion downstairs.

I'm sure Carlos would have complied if I had told him what I wanted, but up to this point, I still hadn't examined myself enough to know what turned me on. Besides, it's hard enough to say the right things in English. I had no idea how to express myself or my desires in Spanish. Sensually, I was lazy. Instead of having to find ways around his explorations, as I had with other boyfriends, or guide him like I had to with Rafiq, I was fine with just lying there in missionary, letting him do his thing. I came to think of my vulva as a hole. The hair and whatever else was down there was merely padding for the pit.

So I learned to define pleasure by the proximity to my lover, not by spasms or tingles or my eyes rolling back in my head. And Carlos, well, he never really noticed anything one way or another. He was too busy enjoying himself.

Carlos and I always spoke in Spanish. I was in Rafiq's shoes now, at the whim of another to help me comprehend long strings of conjugated verbs I'd probably once studied but had long ago forgotten. Though it was frustrating at first, I found that in a new language, I could take on a different persona. Nothing seemed as serious in a language I only half knew. I disconnected from my uncontrollable ambition and felt liberation in the practice of getting absolutely nothing done. I began tie-dyeing and selling T-shirts. I spent the rest of my time working for fifty cents an hour at a coffee shop named Pi, about eighty stairs down the street.

I met a regular there named Noam. He was constantly on the road, traveling all over the world for work, but was based in the United States. I'd hand-press his espresso as we talked about everything from the destruction of the Amazon to the marketplace's best juice stall. (I avoided the one with the freshly cut bull testicles drying above the water bucket.) Noam's voice was so deep that it seemed to make the coffee cups clatter, but also so gentle that it sent shivers up and down my spine. One time, our attraction had caused us to unconsciously lean toward each other. Our lips were about to touch when we were interrupted by a religious procession; a throng of people carried a crucified Jesus down the street. The bloody Jesus reminded me of sinning, and sinning reminded me that the mouth coming at me was the wrong one. I was dating Carlos. Noam's and my lips quickly backtracked into our own separate air space. Though we never hooked up, I had a feeling that our paths would cross later on.

By four months into my stay, I'd become completely content with my daily routine. I'd pump out espressos, have a *choclo con queso* (corn and cheese) in the plaza, consistently get stomachaches from home-brewed *chicha* (fermented corn beer), and make guacamole feasts with Peru's head-sized *paltas* (avocado). The fundamental human things—eating, dancing, sleeping, and screwing—became the most important because there were no external pressures to tell us that we were only as valuable as what we'd accomplished. In that small town, it seemed you were just as good as anyone else as long as you were a good person. In a sense, I'd lost all my will to move up in the world. I felt that maybe moving up, as I had grown to recognize it, was actually moving down; high salaries and occupational titles meant nothing if you couldn't be happy. Then one day while I was serving a latte, my parents called me and told me that I'd gotten in to journalism school. I hesitated for an instant. Maybe I didn't want that anymore. I'd never been more carefree.

I decided I didn't want it.

"Mara," said my mom, "are you kidding me?"

And with that, with those simple words, I was rewired. I immediately fell back to the American standard, where benchmarks for success are the number of letters after a name or digits in a salary. I packed up my bags and got all colonial on Carlos, imposing my ideals on him. I told him what was best for me—going to school—was also best for him. I coerced him to go back to Argentina and enroll in university. We traveled on a bus for two days to make it all the way to Buenos Aires. We stayed in a small apartment with his father, who had lost everything—his huge house, his kids' college accounts—in the economic crisis.

I stayed for two weeks. Carlos took me around his city, but most of the time we stayed in the apartment listening to music and drinking maté—maté with milk, maté with dried orange peel, maté with a dash of espresso on top. The closer my departure date came, the closer we became. Things I could never say in English— I love you—I could say to him in Spanish—*te quiero*—because it felt like I was living in a fantasy world, almost like it all wouldn't count when I got back home. I had so many connotations linked to the English words, but in Spanish the words were free of previous emotional charge.

When I left, I cried a puddle into his sweater. Drops hung from his lashes, but I was ready to get serious again. I was disappointed in myself for how little I'd achieved while I was gone.

WIRED, UNWIRED, AND THEN REWIRED AGAIN

BAT WINGS

We've lived together for more than a quarter century, my vulva and me, but I've never looked at it directly. Betty and all the how-to-get-your-orgasm books said that checking it out is step one. It's amazing how easy it has been to avoid a part of my own body. Maybe I can blame it on evolution. Ever notice how every orifice in the body is strategically placed so it's almost impossible to look into directly? Men are practically born with a dick in their hands, but imagine the cavewoman. If she wanted to see anything, she had to check out her pussy's reflection in a lake.

Maybe if I had been born in second-century China—when a snatch was referred to by such pleasing terms as "The Jewel Terrace," "The Golden Lotus," and "The Open Peony Blossom"—I'd have had a better handle on things. But, I mean, American girls grow up playing with Barbie dolls, who don't even have a "down there" to talk about. Barbie has no labia, no nipples, and no messy pubic hair. She'll never have an untimely queef or smell like anything other than fresh polyethylene, and Ken will never get a pubic hair stuck in his teeth.

I needed some tools for my inspection: a bubble bath, some candles for atmosphere, and a mirror. I set up an exploration zone in my room. I wanted it to feel special.

I hopped in a bubble bath. The bubbles crackled in my ears and I sucked them up my nostrils. The point of the bath was to relax me so I could acquaint myself with my body and prepare myself for scrutiny. I didn't mind being naked, but I just, you know, didn't look down *there*. I gave a little rinse, a scrub, and then I was out, back to sudsing up the extremities. I tried to focus, but like with sex, I found my mind running toward impertinent things, like whether or not wireless radiation can permeate porcelain tubs.

I towel-dried. I used Q-tip after Q-tip until my ear canals were raw. (I know it's bad, but it feels so good.) I went into my room and stood on a blanket. I looked at my reflection from head to toe. I didn't know what had happened; I used to be naked all the time.

Before I turned ten, my nuclear family was almost constantly naked. We lived the life of a small-scale nudist colony, swimming naked, reading naked, watching TV naked, playing naked Parcheesi and naked Connect Four. My parents didn't even believe in pajamas, and especially not underwear, during the nighttime hours. For them it was a conspiracy by the undergarment industry. Elastic leg holes were prone to cut off blood flow to the developing brain.

Even in later years, I was known to skinny dip on occasion, and there are probably pictures of me somewhere, hopefully undeveloped, choreographing the construction of pyramids built out of the bodies of unclothed friends. It's when intimacy is involved that the problem occurs. Mass nudity is a blanket of skin, whereas two people interacting, or even just me alone, takes on deeper meaning somehow.

I did a one-eighty in the mirror, appraising myself. I'd be set if I were just two butt cheeks scooting around town, since when I look at my gluteus, I'm proud. *I made that!* But alas, I'm connected to all sorts of other problematic extremities.

The boobs are a bit too small. When I was younger, I theorized that maybe mammaries were like fish and would grow to the size of their aquarium. But I eventually realized I'd never be anything more than an A-cup girl in a B-cup bra. My jowls are a little too large; they invite pinches. I'd like more of a curve from shoulders to hips. Something a bit more concave would be nice from sternum to waistline. I wish my biceps were thinner than my forearms and my forearms half the size they already are. My legs resemble pythons in the middle of digesting a guinea pig—that's how tumorous my calves are.

So pretty much, I'd like to cut myself in half and stuff the scraps into my bra.

Now here's a real downer: Fiona and I pierced our nipples when we were eighteen. I took the piercings out a couple years later, but the poor things never did completely regain their former structure. (I worry that if I ever breed, the milk flow from an extra two spigots will either drown my offspring or turn them into obese diabetic lumps of flesh held together by onesies.)

And then there's the fact that I have hairy-olas. You know what I'm talking about—not a lion's mane or anything, just a little hair here and there around the nipple region. I was traumatized when I was listening to *Loveline* one night. Adam Carolla took a call from a heinous man who condemned his lover's nipple tresses. I know we're mammals, and I know mammals have hair, but for some reason hair is such a ghastly thing for a woman to bear. I ritualistically pluck out each and every five of them (okay, six of them) every other Wednesday night, cursing each follicle as it falls to the floor.

I conducted my fat tests: I arched my back to see how much flub would fold over. Just one rung: acceptable. I prodded the region where my handful of tits met my armpits and investigated whether or not an intermediate flab boob was developing. With both my hands, I pushed my belly fat together, and then quickly let go. That was a bad idea.

It was finally time to check out the juncture, see what all this flower whoop-de-do was about. I grabbed the two outer lips with forefinger and thumb and then pulled them apart.

I looked.

Then I looked at my face in the mirror.

I recognized that face. That's how I looked when I went to the bathroom to gag after I found out the carnita tacos at one of my parents' nursery parties were actually made from my brother's pet pig, Bob.

No. No. This definitely was not normal. Something was wrong with Clitty Rose. It didn't look anything like a flower. It didn't look like a shell. It didn't look like a fig. It wasn't Greek Modern or Arabian Chic. After I saw Clitty Rose, I understood why I had not paid more attention to it. How had Georgia O'Keeffe gotten away with her pudendal depictions? Her labial floral aesthetics had monopolized vulva symbology for more than half a century, and for this?

Feminist propaganda, that's what all that flower talk was.

Why don't we call it what it really is: an inside-out bat flying backward.

ONE YEAR IN BANGKOK MAKES AN
ANORGASMIC FORGET SHE HAS A COOTER

After Peru, my crotch didn't have a moment to stir for an entire year. I was busy getting my master's in journalism at Columbia and I was serious about getting somewhere. I imagine that had I bothered checking between my legs during that time, my womanhood would have atrophied, almost wilted away. When I graduated, I didn't even have time to think of diddling. I shipped off immediately to Bangkok, Thailand, where I'd been hired as a feature reporter.

The year that followed managed to totally screw up any possibility of orgasm—and not only because I didn't have any sex. Sexually, I regressed in Bangkok. The city is crazy, or maybe it's not and it just made *me* crazy. At any rate, I discovered that a lot of those Bangkok stereotypes and rumors you hear are true, which somehow caused me to have a yearlong dry spell, become asexual, and learn to pay for human contact.

It didn't take long to discover that my twenty-fourth year of life was going to be a lonely one. My editor was originally from New

York. He had run a smut magazine in the States for two years, and rumor had it that he had lived in a tent in a Hawaiian national park smoking Maui Wowie for seven years before moving to Bangkok. His Thai wife left him to go West. He wanted to stay East. He was busy trying to find another Thai woman to take the last one's place. I asked why Thai. "Thai women are more fun!" he said. Another man, who'd been in the country for twenty-seven years, seconded this opinion right away: "Oh, yes, much more fun!" (Through my travels, I've found there are two types of people who leave their home countries: those who are adventurers, and those who don't fit in where they came from. I'll let you decide which type I ran into most.)

More fun? More fun than what, a Jewish five-footer from the States?

At least the monks walking around town with their bald heads and maroon robes saw all us ladies the same—they weren't allowed to touch any of us. Every pussy possessor was equally dirty, no matter what color, creed, or country.

Thailand is proud of its legacy. It's the only Asian country that has never been colonized. They say they praise *sanuk*, having fun, over all else. If it's not *sanuk*, it's not worth the time. It's also the "land of smiles"; that's what they say in all the tourism commercials. They especially pushed that slogan after the tsunami: We smile even when there's a massive tragedy. And it's totally true. The smile is the go-to facial expression, but a smile can mean many different things—think Eskimos and how they supposedly have a gazillion words for snow. As I lunged toward a translator who helped me with my first story, my arms open wide to give her a hug of gratitude, she gave me a beautiful beaming smile while her eyes bugged out of their slits, and she hopped back so far she almost got run over by a careening *tuk tuk*. I found out touching is a no-no, unless it is paid for; instead, the *wai*, a slight bow, is the proper way to say thank you.

I had trouble making friends. Many of the reporters at the paper already had lives there, and some new foreign reporters had coupled among themselves. One girl, who was in a similar situation to mine—single, white, female—was so happy and consistently toothache-sweet that when I spoke to her, I'd turn into a plasticized version of me to be sure I wouldn't burst her bubble. She lasted three months before repatriating herself. (I also carried around a yellow purse from Oaxaca that smelled like wet animal every time it got drenched, which couldn't have helped with the friendships, since it rained a lot.) For my part, I put each and every molecule in my body toward work. Which is what I do best, I suppose.

When touching didn't seem like a possibility, touching became what I wanted. The only epidermal contact I experienced for weeks on end was my own thighs sticking together in the humidity. I had to get some touch from something besides my own lipidinous flabbery. One way was sidling up against one of the men who ran the motorcycle taxis, which was fun in its own reckless close-call-swerving-in-between-traffic-jams kind of way, but each ride also infused my respiratory system with two cigarette packs' worth of smoke—the smog from buses' exhaust pipes reached out and licked passersby like a thick hot tongue.

A Thai massage, I thought, would be perfect for some contact. I went to a place right next to my apartment. There was a sign: snooker, karaoke, and Thai massage. Inside, there was a big window; behind it was a gaggle of girls playing cards, all wearing pants that fit like body paint. Their skin looked as bronzed and smooth as ladies who'd been airbrushed in Neutrogena face-wash commercials. The situation was peculiar. My brain buzzed the same way it had when I cheated on my high school Spanish exams—like I was going to get caught at something. But I didn't know how it all worked yet, so I didn't want to judge. I picked out the girl with #8 pinned to her shirt and everyone cheered—smiles of every different kind were abundant. In a small musty room, she climbed all over me like I was a jungle gym. It was at the moment when she stood on my thighs, pulled my chest up by lifting my arms, and twisted me to the left until my back cracked at least ten times that the men's fetish with Thai women started making sense. She waited on the edge of the bed as I prepared to dress. Why wouldn't she leave? I turned toward the other wall as I pulled my shirt over my head. She smiled and laughed. I counteracted all that good cheer with a sneer; I wanted my privacy. Later I asked a colleague what that was all about.

"They had numbers on? You picked her out of a window?" he asked. "She was probably waiting to see if you wanted a happy ending. That was a brothel."

"Oh," I said. "Yeah, of course." And that's when I really became aware of the sex industry.

The way I perceived Bangkok might say more about me than it does about the place. When I wasn't working, I felt drawn to Bangkok's seedy side. Like looking into the toilet after a good bowel movement, the sex trade both fascinated and repulsed me. I'd go to Soi Nana and Patpong, the two most popular districts for hookers and strip bars in the city. There were other activities—I could have gone to museums, malls, or parks—but my perverse fascination drew me in, and my repulsion kept me there. I believed the sex industry ruled everyone's mind, when in fact, it ruled mine. It was a downward spiral. But in a place so thick with orgasms, I was the farthest from them that I'd ever been.

When I saw women reduced to a commodity, to body parts, to an exchange of a chunk of change left after a night out drinking, the practice confirmed everything I'd feared was true. Men didn't want a brain, didn't want a companion. They wanted a female they could purchase, control, and boil down to one-way terms. There, men finally felt like the king of the mountain because they could buy a hot young chick for the same price they used to pay for a McDonald's Happy Meal. I got so, so jaded by stories I heard. A man keeping a Thai girl on retainer while he had his family in the States, for instance.

When the man touched the girl, her personality didn't matter anymore; she disappeared and became only an empty body. The more I saw men interacting and making transactions for purely physical ends, the more I disengaged from my own body and transferred all my being toward my mind. I kept myself safe. I became a brain preserved in a glass jar.

I know people can get screwed in the crossfire of these sweeping generalizations. In Bangkok, I knew biracial couples who truly loved each other, and not because either one was bought. I also had a friend who told me his Thai girlfriend was propositioned by another male right in front of him; this man had suspected that all Thai women with white men were prostitutes.

Bangkok was the opposite of India; I was as invisible to the men there as a piece of lint on someone's sock. It was the Thai women everyone was after. I was so ignored, I began to forget I was a girl. All my life I'd taken my femininity for granted—in India, I had even tried to hide it—but now it felt like it was something transitory, like a fine layer of perfume that I'd accidentally washed off. So much of my identity was built on the reflection I saw in others' reactions. I longed for the moments I used to hate, the objectifying catcalls when some dude on the sidewalk would snicker, suck his teeth, make obscene comments, or blow kisses in the air. At least when that happened, I knew I was there.

It didn't help that the Thai people often referred to women by "sir" in English. It wasn't their fault, it's just the way the pronouns got translated, but I couldn't help but get frustrated. When I threatened them with bared teeth and yelled, "I'm not a SIR!" they'd give me one of the smiles in their repertoire, the one that said, *Get this crazy* farang *away from me.* "It's ma'am! MA'AM! Get it straight!" If I had had the balls, I would have dropped my pants and showed them my cooter right there. (Wait, that's not right—balls, cooter—but you get the point.)

Every girl there was so tiny that even though I was a size four, petite by U.S. standards, I felt like a Snuffleupagus among a herd of My Little Ponies. When I rummaged through the fashions at clothing shops, the proprietors would look me up and down and then say, with a smile but a don't-you-dare-stretch-that-out look in their eyes, "No large!" So I kind of went mildly anorexic for a year. I soaked up nutrition as I roamed the streets, inhaling the fumes from frying pans sizzling with greens and garlic, fresh chilies mashed in a mortar and pestle singeing my nostrils, much as the pungent smell of piss in India had. Don't be misguided, as I was: Not eating doesn't change your bone structure from sturdy Eastern European peasant–like to more sylphlike; it only makes you lose your hair.

Let me tell you about one of the only times in the entire year that a man made a pass at me. I went to a male sex show with my gay Thai friend. I was the only girl in the audience made up of whooping men. The boys stood on the stage with little jockey pants on, all bright colors like a fancy string of Christmas lights. They had numbers pinned close to their bulging groins and strutted around presenting their "packages" before the real acrobatics began, which included cock-in-butt contortions I never could have fathomed, even if I'd made sodomy the subject of my master's thesis. After the show, the Thai boys, who made most of their money by prostituting themselves to the gay spectators, excitedly streamed off the stage to greet me—their one chance at scoring a girl. Weirdly enough, by that point, their advances, though they were only for money, felt oddly validating. But I had to pass on the opportunity. Call me uptight, but I have this thing about venereal diseases: I don't want one. Instead, I continued my weekly massages for my quota of human contact. I'd found a new place where there were bright lights and no numbers pinned to the girls' jeans.

At one point, Fiona came to visit me. Both of us were having a rough time. She'd just broken up with someone and was dating someone new. But the problem was with her agents in New York: They had just told her to lose her cherubic cheeks. Apparently casting directors weren't looking for ingenues who didn't have an implosion on either side of their faces. She wasn't sure how to go about doing that since there wasn't necessarily a way to go on a diet from the neck up, and the rest of her body was already up-to-their-standard lithe. While I starved myself and she worked out, we pondered the fucked-up cultural norms and pressures that said thin was divine. She decided to cut those agents, along with that last boyfriend, out of her life.

Soon after Fiona left, I became sick of fighting against what seemed to be the prevailing attitude; I distanced myself from what was going on and viewed it all like an absurdist comedy. That's when I finally made two friends: Gavin from England and Pete from the States. They both exhibited the attitude I'd hated and feared, but by that point I'd become immune to it all. I gave in. I joined in. I refused to let it affect me anymore.

I'd go to the go-go bars with Gavin and Pete. We'd ride the mechanical bull over happy hour Chang Beers. I'd watch women open bottles with their vulvas and shoot Ping-Pong balls and darts out of them. Sure, I was disgusted, especially when the Ping-Pong ball had me in its trajectory. But I couldn't help wondering if things would be different for me if I had the chutzpah to jam one of those up there and had strong enough pubococcygeus muscles to launch it into the air.

Gavin and Pete both taught school and gave me a window into the expat male world. They'd often pick up prostitutes after a long night out on the town. After years there, they were desensitized, and paying was the norm. When we met up with their other friends at bars, we might slip into the conversation at the point where one might be saying, ". . . and that's when I decided that I would never have sex with a ladyboy again." They related stories of getting chlamydia tests (which often came out positive) the old-fashioned way, with a cotton swab down the head. Afterward, we'd go out for a beer to help subdue the pain.

Gavin wanted to go back to England, but he was worried about what people would say. If he told anyone he'd been in Bangkok for three years, he knew what they'd think. I had to agree.

"But I don't want them to think that," he said. "How will I get a date?"

I asked him why he did it, then. "It's too easy here," he said. "Everything, it's all handed to you on a silver tray."

My brothers soon came for a weeklong visit. Without thinking, I got Gavin and Pete to lead us on an excursion to all the best go-go bars. There were palaces, the famous reclining Buddha, and museums, too, but no: I had begun thinking that women were all that men wanted to see. We went to one club where women in schoolgirl uniforms but no underwear danced on the floor above a translucent ceiling, so when they ground against the floor, everyone on the floor below got to know them *very* well. One girl got especially attached to my brother, and I started cheering them on. I was telling him he could have my apartment for the night. I'd gone completely loony. I thought that was the only way he'd have fun.

"Mara, what's wrong with you?" he asked. "You're getting scary."

Meanwhile, Fiona called me to say she'd broken up with that last someone and was now with Pedro. He even liked to eat raw food, which was her current modus operandi. She was going to get married after knowing him not even two months.

That's when I told her she could always get a divorce.

By that point, see, I couldn't have gotten much more cynical about relationships. But just like that, Fiona continued to stay ahead of me, and at twenty-four, she became a wife.

I guessed she'd soon be nesting, so there went my post-Bangkok pullout couch.

While I reported on breaking cultural phenomena for the newspaper like clothes for fat girls and the launch of booze cruises down the Chao Phraya River, my employer began sponsoring protests against the then Prime Minister, Thaksin Shinawatra. The Thaksin supporters lined up outside of our office to protest. One time a small pipe bomb exploded in our front yard, though it made nothing more than a divot in our foliage. Then a group of thugs smothered one of our nearby offices with eleven bags of pig feces. I think by this point I'd become rather nihilistic. I kept hoping for bombs, for chaos, for destruction. Maybe I just wanted an excuse to call all my friends in the United States and say, "Yeah, don't worry about me, I'm fine," or maybe I just wanted a distraction, something to blow me out of the reality I'd chosen to live in.

In any case, I quit. But I wasn't ready to go home.

During a story I had reported earlier in the year, I'd met a man who worked with Karen refugees from Burma. His organization concerned itself with education. He'd make dangerous journeys into the Karen state to disseminate textbooks and curriculum to ethnic minorities displaced by Myanmar's military junta. (Although Myanmar is the country's official name, many continue to call it Burma because the population was never given a chance to vote on the change.) Since I was out of a job, he invited me up north to Mae Sariang, near Thailand's border with Burma, to teach one of the Karen how to be a journalist. My student quickly came up with a loving nickname for me, Naw La Uh, which she told me translated to Ms. Ugly.

Mae Sariang was a beautiful place. It refreshed me. It even gave me the most action I had all year: my bicycle and me, bumping along a snaking canal, my hair blowing in the wind and my crotch finally getting some play.

I pushed middle-aged men and their prostitutes to the back of my mind; the Karen put things into perspective for me. They've had to deal with things that most of us are lucky enough never to have to think about and don't have the imagination to conjure. When I was visiting one of the refugee camps, it was quite common to hear someone say, "I was lucky, only my husband and brother were killed." One of these victims had a picture of the WTC Twin Towers in mid-collapse taped up on her thin bamboo wall. She told me she loved the United States and was so excited because she knew one day they'd come to Burma and fight for freedom and democracy. I wanted to cry—and, finally, not for myself.

After sharing life with the Karen for a month, I was curious to see what Burma was about. On my second day in the country, I met a guy from the States named Dr. Reynolds who worked for an international aid organization. He was an earthy dude with frizzy cropped blondish hair and a gangly body. And despite being more than six feet tall, more than a foot taller than I am, he still managed to look me in the eyes. He actually saw me.

I had been living in a place where you couldn't escape sexuality, whereas where he'd lived for the past year, even shorts could be considered lewd. Somehow, those two extremes allowed us to meet in the middle. We went out on a date in Yangon, the capital city. He bought some boiled peanuts from a street vendor; I mashed them into a ball and then pushed a smiley face design into the lump. That was how deeply I'd regressed. I was acting like a kindergartener who had a crush and thought I'd impress him by playing with my paste. I guess it worked, though, because we were soon zooming over to his house—just a few blocks from Aung San Suu Kyi, the pro-democracy activist, who'd been under house arrest for more than a decade.

Dr. Reynolds leaned in to kiss me. I puckered up, getting ready. It would have been my first kiss in more than a year, and I was more than ready. Leaning, leaning, leaning, leaning . . . and then I wasn't there anymore. I freaked out. I couldn't handle the newfound intimacy that year had taught me to live without. I scooted myself to the furthest reaches of his sofa and stared at him like a kid who'd lost her parents in the grocery store. He remained calm while trying to coax my id off the ceiling and my libido from its place of hiding. My heart was pounding from fear. If he wanted my body, then surely that meant he'd be leaving my mind behind, right? His touch would make me disappear.

Poor guy, he didn't realize over the boiled peanuts and beer that later he would have a lunatic in his living room. It's just that the whole idea of sexual attraction to me, by that point, was as foreign as the fried locust snacks I'd had during my first week in Southeast Asia. As he drove me to my hostel, I was flushed with embarrassment. Aung San Suu Kyi was an unwilling prisoner in her own country while I'd willingly checked myself into a cell of my own.

"Sorry," I said. I slammed the car door quickly, not wanting to hear what he was going to say next.

After a couple days, we met up again. I think his deprivation ran as deeply as mine did because somehow he was able to overlook my quirks and patiently reacquaint me to the world of physical interaction. Again, as in Cuzco, things moved quickly. We ditched all foreplay—unless you call him palpating my belly and checking my blood pressure foreplay (he was a doctor after all; I had to take advantage). You'd think all those Ping-Pong-ball visuals would have gotten me in touch, but I'd grown completely estranged from my body—had disowned it, in a way—and when I got into his bed, I guess you could say I went consciously unconscious. I didn't feel much, but feeling wasn't the main goal at the time. I was happy just to be reminded I was a female.

I continued to visit him regularly during my monthlong Burma stay. I was in awe of human contact. I felt like I had an empty battery that could only be charged up through touch.

With Dr. Reynolds still on my mind, I flew back to Bangkok to pack up. It turned out that my friend Gavin had had a mishap while I was away. Because much of the Internet is censored in Burma, he wasn't able to contact me. He had bought a woman for the night and woken up three days later with a smashing headache and a lot of extra space on his shelf—no more computer, I-Pod, DVD player, or stereo. As I finally left Bangkok for good, I gifted him a Ganesha statue, the Hindu god who's said to remove obstacles, to watch over affairs of the mattress. I didn't necessarily like his use of prostitutes, but I still cared about him and wanted him to get screwed regularly.

Upon my return home to San Diego, I tried to figure out my next logical career step, but in the meantime, I got a waitress job at Olive Garden. One of the highlights of the job was receiving, along with my tip, a psychotherapist's business card with a personal note: *If you'd like, please call.* I washed and tumble-dried it along with my Alfredo-stained apron until all the words had rubbed off.

ONE YEAR IN BANGKOK

I began looking for a job in journalism, and the *Village Voice* took particular interest. Within three months of returning home and becoming quite savvy in the ways of shaving Romano cheese over pastas, I moved to New York City to become a staff writer at the alt-weekly.

Throughout my time at home, I'd managed to stay in touch with Dr. Reynolds. He'd also moved back to the States. We visited each other twice. I was comfortable living an expensive airplane ticket apart. It meant I wouldn't have to break many of my barriers or allocate my could-be-working time toward building a relationship, yet I could still have someone to call up and could fool myself into believing I was age-appropriate in my dealings with intimate partnerships. But by month three in New York, we'd both become consumed by our respective careers and talked less and less, until we didn't talk at all. I began channeling all my sexual energies into the printed page, but I soon became aware of my pattern of sex-focused articles (by way of other people, somewhat embarrassingly, pointing it out). My stories were getting a whole lot more action than I was, and at twenty-six, I realized I was just as sexually clueless about myself as I had been at eighteen. Shit!

BREATH JUNKIE

"It's certainly a flower!" Fiona said. "It's a lily. It's like a beautiful crimson orchid. It is."

I couldn't convince Fiona. O'Keeffe had already infected her brain. She went on to tell me that I should do a nude photo shoot like she had done so that I could appreciate my body. I could see myself through an artist's eyes, she said. I told her she was insane for posing nude. "You know what happens to girls whose nudie pics are posted on the Internet," I said.

"I'm not ashamed," she said. "They're beeeaaautiful."

She said "beautiful" all drawn out like it was a rubber band; the more she stretched the word, the more power it would have by the last syllable. Not that a "beautiful" stretched two minutes long would do anything to change what people would say when they got their hands on her nudie pics. "Pornography," that's what they would say.

One hundred years ago, all this orgasm stuff wasn't such an issue. Female sexuality hardly seemed to matter. I read about it in

Rachel Maines's book *The Technology of Orgasm*. At the slightest signs of anxiety, sleeplessness, irritability, nervousness, erotic fantasy, or vaginal lubrication, I would have been taken to a doctor. He would have diagnosed me with hysteria, brought me into his vibratory "operating theater"—for a fee, of course—and manually massaged or used a "therapeutic appliance" on my vulva until I reached "hysterical paroxysm," at which point I would have been cured.

Unfortunately, the American Psychiatric Association took hysteria off their list of disorders in 1952. I suppose it's a good thing that female arousal is no longer seen as an illness, but I do wonder: would health insurance have covered that?

Now there are all these orgasms to choose from—many more than I ever could have imagined. There is the clitoral orgasm crowd, which includes the clitcentric Granny of Masturbation. To her, planet clit revolves around the orgasm sun. Then there is the post-porn modernist Annie Sprinkle, a close friend of Betty's who believes orgasm can be expanded to a whole bodily galaxy (I hear they always get into fights about this). She had sex with 3,500 people in ten years, part research and part fun, and says that though each female orgasm is as unique as a grain of sand, they can be broken up into seven categories: dream-gasms, microgasms, inter-vaginal orgasms, breath and energy orgasms, clitoral orgasms, combination-gasms, and megagasms—the last of which are so potent, she says, that they may require an "orgasm midwife" to deliver. She documented a five-minute megagasm in her film *Sluts and Goddesses* and said people in her presence experienced empathetic microgasmic aftershocks.

I felt like I had to take baby steps; I couldn't ask for a megagasm right away. Plus, I wanted a break from vaginas, so I went to a workshop on Tantric energy orgasms held by Barbara Carrellas, a sex educator and Urban Tantric practitioner. She said we'd be having orgasms by the end of two hours without unbuttoning anything; vaginas would be of no use for this orgasm, which, for the time being, I felt was a good thing. Baby steps.

"The human experience is erotic" was the first thing she told us.

Barbara somehow seemed like the embodiment of an orgasm as one might appear at a Grateful Dead concert. She was dressed in electric tie-dye of pinks and oranges, including strips of hot pink interspersed throughout her blond hair, and she wore thick oval-framed glasses.

She called herself a sexual expansionist and said anything could be sex if it had sexual intention behind it. She was pissed off at Bill Clinton, a sexual reductionist, for saying an office blow job wasn't sex. I found out many lesbians felt this way, because if sex were defined only as a penis entering a vagina, then all lesbians would inherently have no sex lives at all. Expanding the definition of sex is an issue of equality.

Barbara set up her stereo in a small lecture room. About sixteen people gathered in a circle. "Most people practice the Mount Saint Helens orgasm," Barbara said, meaning they clench all their muscles and have a small unsatisfying explosion at a low peak. From childhood, they learn to practice masturbation clandestinely. "Don't breathe, shut up, come fast" is how it usually goes, she said: people get into the habit and don't know how to change. She said breathing changes consciousness and could lead to an ecstatic state: "You'll be stranded somewhere in between the earth and the moon."

Everyone stared at Barbara gape-eyed as she lay in the mush pot of our circle. She began rocking her pelvis forward. She was giving a demonstration of the Clench and Hold Energy Orgasm. She took deep breaths. "The most erotic tool is the breath," she said. "It's even more important than a vibrator. Most people breathe barely enough to survive." She said it was important to disperse sexual energy throughout the body by deep breathing—before coming —because it'd lead to a full-body experience.

"You want to fill a whole five-gallon jug with energy," she said, meaning the whole body, "instead of a little coffee cup." She cupped her crotch to show where the coffee cup was.

As she rocked, her arms spiraled like windmills and she began Kegeling. "It brings energy up from the furnace," she said, grabbing her crotch again. Barbara seemed incapable of embarrassment, but some people in the circle began to giggle uncomfortably. She breathed into her chakras, which are centers of spiritual power within the body. Each chakra is linked to a different sound, she said. If you're not orgasming yourself, you can listen to your neighbors and play "guess where the orgasm is." It's deep and resonating when close to the genitals and becomes higher and higher until it's practically a screech at the top of the head—she sounded like the fingers on a piano do, when sliding the keys from left to right, as her body seesawed. Her arms flailed. She breathed, arched, and shuddered.

It was quite a sight; Barbara was having the most amazing orgasm in the most unromantic surroundings—the middle of a fluorescent-lit lecture room—with all her clothes on. I thought she had to be acting, but that's one of her techniques. She says fake it until you feel it. She clenched all her muscles and took three final big breaths. Then she held her breath. When she released, she squirmed like she had ants in her pants—or dynamite.

Barbara turned to us and said, "Your turn." Six people had already deserted the mission. The rest of us lay down and started breathing. "Concentrate on the breath and moving energy," said Barbara. "These tools give your mind erotically constructive things to do instead of worrying and losing focus during sex. Stay with your body." She walked around us and talked us into our trance. "Imagine nice, juicy molten red from the center of the earth moving through your body," she said. "Throw a Kegel in there when you can."

I breathed in and blew out like I was trying to put out a raging fire. *This* I could do; I could breathe. But fuck, my hands started tingling. A groaning and moaning symphony played in stereo from the surround-sound mouths all about me. I refused to join in. I felt silly making sounds. Barbara told us to envision building an eggshell out of brilliant colors and erotic energies around our heaving bodies.

"Keep breathing!"

Twenty minutes later:

My lips turned to stone. I couldn't move them. Pressure developed in my chest. "Clench!" she yelled. The moans around me ceased. There were just small, constipated grunts here and there. "Release!" she said. My body felt warm and prickly, like I'd landed on a bed of baby cacti. My lips spasmed, and my eyeballs twitched. I felt dizzy, queasy, lightheaded, and weak.

"If you do that during sex," she said smiling, hovering above a carpet of jerking bodies, "you'll never be disappointed in your orgasmic response."

No offense to Barbara—I mean, it felt neat and all—but seriously: that couldn't be an orgasm. That was hyperventilation.

SKELETON

Rori, my therapist, wore her knee-high boots with a skirt hem hovering about four inches above; she drank her Diet Snapples as I spewed tales. She said there was no tear limit, in therapy or in life. You can cry forever; there's always another box of tissues in the closet. But I wouldn't do it. I wouldn't cry. Every time I felt a tingle in my throat, I'd stop myself by changing the subject.

By this time around, I was still trying to demonstrate the extent of my inadequacies, trying to show her enough wrong with me to warrant my orgasmic difficulties. So I told her about my first job. It was at a Baskin-Robbins ice cream parlor. I told her how my boss, at thirty-two years old, was twice my age. I laughed when I told her this because I often liked to pretend that potentially traumatic things were actually funny. It was part of the no-capital-letters game Keena had taught me: nothing's a big deal if you don't make it one.

My boss was married. He stood behind me one night when I was mopping. He said I was doing it wrong. He wanted to show me how to do it right. Then he took me in his car to a place I didn't recognize even though I'd lived in the area my whole life. It was dark. My contact popped out; half my vision was blurry. He gave me some statistics; he told me seventy-five percent of spouses cheat. He asked me if I wanted to help him join the majority. I said, "No, please."

For months, I had dreams that men were hiding in the back of my car. I made friends accompany me everywhere.

As I told Rori all this, I wasn't laughing anymore, but I wasn't about to cry. I hadn't cried about this since the night it happened. He hadn't raped me; the whole episode, though disillusioning, wasn't worth tears.

"It's okay to feel," she said.

And that's when my eyes started dripping. They wouldn't stop. If the human body was mostly water, I feared I'd cry until I was nothing but bones.

SKELETON

THE MONK WHO KNOWS PUSSY

There's one person in the city who always makes me feel better, and he's at the Union Square Greenmarket.

On my way to see him, I passed a woman whose shopping bag said Shoe-Gasm—yet another kind of gasm that was eluding me. I meandered through the many vegetable stalls, eyeing the goods; it looked like the perfect season for phallic produce. The mound of zucchinis reminded me of Betty. I still hadn't bought that vibrator—and fuck, the Kegels! I had forgotten the Kegels. So I ferociously Kegeled, making up for lost pubococcygeus workout time, as I made my way over to the Muffin Madness stall, where Atman sells his vegan baked goods. He's only available from seven a.m. until five p.m. Wednesdays and Fridays; otherwise he's in his upstate ashram. I used to visit him after rough days of reporting at the *Voice*. He always had answers, even if I didn't have questions, and because his accent is so heavy, I had to intuitively interpret half of his advice anyway, which somehow led to a healthy dose of introspection.

It was as if Atman were magically beamed from his hometown in Punjab into some urban accountant's after-work leisure outfit. His skin is the color of his bran muffins, which are sweetened with locally made apple juice, and his more-pepper-than-salt hair pokes out the sides of his baseball cap.

When I lived in India, I mocked the people who went there on a spiritual guru hunt. I figured spirituality, if you yearned for it, wouldn't come from crossing an ocean to a place you didn't understand. So I couldn't exactly comprehend why I was going to a male Indian monk at an organic muffin stand in the middle of New York City to help me figure out my own crotch.

But reason couldn't stop me. I picked up my scone—my culinary therapy—as he kissed me on the cheek. I whispered in his ear, "Can I talk to you about something?"

I told Atman about my circumstances—the orgasm, the book, everything.

"About your flower?" he yelled. "You're writing about your flower!"

He thought it was a flower too? The feminists obviously had a good campaign going with this flower nonsense. But I didn't want to fight with a guru.

"Yeah, my flower," I said. "Any advice?"

"Your flower is like the mother," he said. "It is the most important thing. This is just the beginning."

This was awkward. People were holding out bills, waiting to buy muffins and cookies. I handed him the money for my scone; he kept talking.

"Why do we wear it tighter down there?" he said, pointing to my crotch. While hungry people were still staring at us, he began telling me that in his ashram, no one wears underwear. "Why tight, tight, tight in these spaces? What is the point? We need the air for breathing."

THE MONK WHO KNOWS PUSSY

I was blushing. I stepped back a little, still holding out the money. *Please just take it already.*

"You have all the tools and blueprint in your intuition," he said, handing me my change. "There's crystal-clear clarity, not to be confused ever. Just remember the fictional touch for the neurological mind."

I had no idea what he was talking about.

"Something practical," he continued. "Spray inside with rose water and sometimes grooming a little bit."

This is actually how Atman talked.

But why did he, a celibate man, know so much about pussy? I shoved the scone down my throat as if the baked good would somehow clog that trajectory of thinking and decided to just accept it. Atman was now officially the guru of my southern hemisphere. He hugged me. "Love, love, love to self."

Though it was strange and almost disconcerting that a monk had just advised me to groom my pussy in front of stroller-wielding moms and their toddlers, the visit left me oddly invigorated. Things started looking up. When I went to work that weekend, I began looking at each bar patron as a palpable expression of orgasm: each person, after all, came from at least one orgasm, if not two. There were walking, talking, dancing, kissing, drinking, retarded orgasms all over the place. Orgasms were giving me tips and spilling beer on me. Even me: I was a cocktailing orgasm.

The vag even lodged itself into my subconscious. I kept having vulva dreams. I was on vacation with my family and we wanted to see this fairy-tale-esque town from above. We hopped inside a flying furry vulva. We soon joined a whole flock of them, and they were all toting foreigners around like *tuk tuks* in Thailand. We moved into V-formation, with my family at the head. As the breeze ripped through my hair, I woke up. I'm still bothered that I don't know how vulvas land, not to mention disturbed that my family took the ride with me.

I stopped differentiating my keys by color. I started identifying the one that opened my front door by the V-shaped divot that reminded me of a crotch. The heavy breathing of Prospect Park joggers and the rhythmic creaking of my ceiling fan started sounding indecent. I couldn't eat a banana in public without thinking I was going to get arrested for lewd behavior with a defenseless fruit. When I asked a friend if she wanted a coffee and she replied, "Yes, black and straight up," I couldn't help but giggle. And I started waking up with Earl the Stuffed Elephant's trunk in my hand even more than usual.

Conclusion: My down there was waking up.

I needed a new channel to shovel all of this newfound arousal into, and unfortunately, a part of me obviously thought a more direct route to orgasm somehow involved male company. The idea had been ingrained in me for more than a quarter century, after all. To hasten the dating process and the ultimate orgasmic goal, I placed my profile on an Internet dating site called Nerve. I had tried Internet dating once before, but I discovered it was as time-consuming as having a job. I ditched it right quick. But now, I kind of felt like dating was allowed to take up time because it was part of my journey. I made my moniker Euphorbia anoplia, the Latin name of the last cactus I killed (its corpse is still rotting on top of my dresser). I felt it was the first step toward embracing my upbringing.

I had a talk with my roommate Leigh, as she was also prowling the Internet. She gave me a New York City dating roundup: guys have to have money, and the girls have to be skinny. "That's why I'm going to the gym," she said as she dashed out the door.

My first date was with a tall guy with curly hair. We both said we liked to people-watch on our profiles—so many people say they like to people-watch on their profiles that the streets must be filled with watchers who watch the watchers watching—but we didn't have much more in common because, before I knew it, I was telling him that I didn't like cats (he had a cat) and that I didn't watch much theater (he's a playwright). All I could think about was how I wanted to take one of his spiraling curls, stretch it out, and watch it spring back into place. The date was over. He wanted my proper e-mail—we had only been communicating via our profile pages—but I dreaded divulging my full name.

The question in the twenty-first century is not *if* but *when* you will be Googled. I had some dating challenges ahead, to say the least, and you're reading the reason why. You can expect that if a date knows your full name, then he also knows how fast you ran the mile in high school, about the fight you had with your psychobiology professor when you left that nasty comment on the class Web board, and what you looked like at your best friend's wedding reception after four hours at an open bar. In my case, my suitors could find something that said: Mara Altman Is Writing a Book About How She Has Never Orgasmed.

Go ahead, Google me.

BLACK BELT

I had an appointment with my pussy. I was just out of the shower and I traipsed over to my room. Tonight was the night; I was finally going to do something about this masturbation stuff. I couldn't—I wouldn't—leave it all up to guys. I'd bought a fresh bottle from the corner wine shop (all the shopkeepers were still cute, and still gay), and I drank it until my senses felt mildly cracked. I thought it was okay to drink alone. I wasn't necessarily alone anyway. I was with Clitty Rose. I looked down at my black triangle, which was as still and steady as a cheetah before pouncing on prey. I took another sip, and then I plunged my hand into my crevasse like I would a clogged sink, apprehensive about discovering the culprit behind the blockage but trying to get the chore done expeditiously. I felt around a bit. Not so terrible, really. Okay, mildly disgusting. Like mushy banana. Innocuous, though, for the most part.

Then my mom called. I shouldn't have answered, but I probably wanted to be distracted. She asked how everything was going. Any relationships to report? I told her I'd just met a guy named Joe on the Internet. I liked him, kind of a lot, I said, but maybe he just thought he'd get me into bed easily because he knew about my book already. "Don't worry," she said. "It'll come."

Then I heard my dad in the background. "And so will she!"

You can't go digging into your crotch after Keena calls, can you? It'd almost be incestuous or something.

Plus, I had things to do anyway. There were always things to do.

Back to Joe. I had met Joe about a week before. We'd already been on a couple dates since then. I was embarrassed about every reaction I had to him. He had almond eyes that locked to mine. His square jaw framed a pucker I could have munched on for hours. He was on the shorter side, and our steps, his arm over my shoulder, my arm around his waist, had a great rhythmic glide. We had so much in common. We were both writers. We both had brown hair, too. But I couldn't tell if he liked me for me or if he just wanted Clitty Rose.

He kissed me all sweetlike on our first date. After we parted, I Googled him. I found his MySpace page and downloaded some songs he'd composed and recorded. I know when I like someone because I get this compulsive urge to communicate. I had to practice a large amount of restraint—Leigh said protocol required that I wait for him to make second contact—so I prepared myself to spend the week listening to my interior monologue tell things to him.

But before the week was over, he called me late—on the cusp of straight-up booty-call hour—and said it was too beautiful a night to waste. He wanted to know if I would be up for a stroll. Leigh would have told me that wasn't good strategy, but she wasn't there, so I said yes. When he arrived on his bicycle, I unconsciously began humming one of his MySpace songs; when I realized it, my eyes bugged out and I turned the rhythm into a squeaky awkward yawn. We meandered to the park and lay on the grass, staring at the moon. It was fall; the leaves were crunchy below. I was so glad when he kissed me because I was sick of pretending I knew what he was talking about when he spoke of Foucault's comparison of society to the Panopticon prison design. I made a mental note to look that up on Wikipedia later on. As we got up to leave, I pulled dead grass from my matted hair and he swatted my arm. It was my ant tattoo; he thought it was crawling toward my elbow.

Shortly after, we ended up in my room. He took off his shirt. With the hemline of my own shirt in his mouth, he bulldozed it up my stomach. I halted the motion at my bra's underwire. I wondered why he was actually there. Was he just horny and couldn't get to sleep? I wanted to enjoy the moment and get all the pleasure out of it, but I couldn't. I started playing defense—I have a black belt in defensive make-out techniques—and blocked his every effort to strip me.

"How do I know I'm not just going to be a chapter in your book," he asked when we sat up. "Or a footnote?"

I couldn't believe he had asked me that. He had contacted me first; he was the one pursuing this relationship.

"How do I know that *you* don't just want to be a chapter in my book?" I said. "Or the guy who gives me my first orgasm?"

We both shrugged. He kissed me again.

"This is the point when everything comes off or it's time to go home," he said.

I walked him out.

IF YOU BUILD A BAR, THEY WILL COME

At the bar, I met a graphic designer who mostly works on fonts. Without any prompting, he told me **Braggadoccio** was the sexiest font because it's big and bold, and when you pronounce it, the lips are left poised for fellatio. Bars put sex on the brain. I don't quite get how the smell of stale alcohol mixed with cheap nostril-biting perfume, the sticky alcohol residue under my shoe, and the auditory nightmare that is dozens of people yelling over one another are such sexy things when occurring simultaneously, but they are. The two three-letter words—"bar" and "sex"—have some sort of symbiotic relationship. They survive off each other. It's also quite possible that sex was just the station I was tuned to. An older tourist couple, who seemed standard in every way when they first sat down in my section, were soon asking me where they could find a third (and maybe even a fourth) to join an orgy. Luckily, this I could help them with. Knowing the answer from my previous job, I brought over a *Village Voice* and opened to the back page escort advertisements, a full menu of people. They loved New York, they said.

Then one day a dude came in just as my shift was ending. He was an older guy, in his mid-fifties, with long thinning hair and a belly protruding at a perpendicular angle. He could easily have perched a beverage and probably even a remote control sturdily on top of it. I started chatting with him, as I would with any customer. Turns out he was the father of one of the bouncers, Bam Bam. Bam Bam was prone to blurting out unappealing comments to the female staff, myself included—things like, "I want to bang you like a piñata" and "Flash me, please." I disregarded his utterances because I knew they were only desperate pleas—like his sleeve of tattoos or overly worked-out body—for passersby to recognize he had a penis hovering somewhere between his bulging thighs. Like the flasher I met when I was ten, Bam Bam wanted people to know how uncomplicated he was. We all knew.

His father was charming, quite unlike his son. He held out his hand and introduced himself as Barry Goldman. He said he was enchanted. As we spoke more, he revealed that he was in the sex business and taught G-spot manipulation and massage as well as BDSM. He said he was known for his monthly foot fetish parties in the city, but he'd also starred in his own sadomasochistic porn videos. Most of the filming took place in his Jersey City home, in a room he called the dungeon.

"I teach couples how to sew up pussies, put needles into breasts," he said, as nonchalantly as the usual bar patron might ask for a Budweiser pitcher. "Stuff like that."

Without a proper response lined up, I went into default mode: "Can I get you a drink?"

He ordered a nonalcoholic beer.

What? I thought two bottles of tequila were prerequisites to sewing up pussies. Shit, two bottles of tequila were prerequisites to just hearing about sewing up pussies.

IF YOU BUILD A BAR, THEY WILL COME

As I went to fetch his beer, I swigged a shot of Jäger. I needed liquid courage. Here was someone who could help me push my boundaries. Our meeting seemed too serendipitous to dismiss. I was intrigued but felt a bit uneasy. As I delivered his beer, I told him about my project and asked him if I could stop by sometime. "I'm just curious is all," I said. "Just curious."

He said orgasms were his forte; he'd even taught some women to be squirters. He said he was patient and would spend a whole day getting a woman nice and stretched out for a fisting.

"Mmm," I said, nodding. "That sounds really kind of you."

He gave me his details and a wink. I looked at the paper when I got off work; it read MASTERS OF PAIN. The only thing I knew about S&M I had learned from a salesman in Thailand who had been re-marketing his excess stock of electrical mosquito swatters as shock-sational spankers. And all he said about it was this: It hurts.

BLINDFOLDS

I put off calling Barry Goldman because Joe was constantly at the top of my to-do list. In spite of the way things had ended last time, we had another date scheduled.

We sat on my fire escape and stroked each other's thighs while we listened to a folksy-type music compilation. He poked my ant tattoo and said, "It looks like it's trying to get somewhere."

Aren't we all, I was thinking.

There was only dark cement below us. My neighbor, The Collector, who obsessively hoards trash on our patio, had just had his heaps of junk picked up the other day. No one had any baggage at the moment; I couldn't imagine it anyway. I wore a bra with no underwire and no tricky gimmicks in the back—no excuses for stopping my tiny tits from flying free when called upon. I wanted to give Joe a little bit more than last time; a little crumb trail to know there was an eventual path to pussy. I'd talked with friends many times, and we had all agreed: A guy wants sex immediately, but if you give it to him too soon, he loses interest. Plus, I wasn't ready. I wanted to be able to have a one-night stand, but I wasn't there yet. I wasn't sure if I'd ever be.

And that bothered me. I didn't think I had to be that way. I'd grown up to believe women's libidos were weaker than men's. All societal messages relay that guys are the ones with the drive and gals have to be the demure ones, the ones holding back those fierce loving machines. I think the propaganda worked in my case; it castrated my concupiscence. If it did that to me, I can only imagine the license it gave men to think with and live by their cum-spurting engines. They're told they have a second brain in their crotch. They're always talking about "thinking with their other head." Imagine if girls heard from the time they hit puberty that their pussy had a brain that could usurp the control from their cranially enclosed one and that they could then blame it for their lapses in judgment.

We landed on the bed and started groping. When I kissed the back of his lobes, he made sweet, breathy noises. He knew exactly what he was doing as he caressed my body, nipped my belly, and twisted my areolas until they turned into two little knots. I tried to emulate his small groans of pleasure as I scouted out the next location on his body to manipulate.

Before this fourth date, I had stopped mining Nerve for other guys. I was hoping Joe would stick. Even in new media, gender roles have managed to hold. A guy pursues with an e-mail, and a girl weeds out who she does and doesn't like. I still checked the site daily for messages and, of course, checked up on Joe as well. I could see he'd been online recently. That was okay. Fine. Lots of cute girls to see and maybe, just maybe, he was checking up on me.

He pulled out a blue-silk sleeping mask and put it over his face. Comets, moons, and stars were outlined in yellow. The border was in black. The music stopped, as if on cue. I had a good excuse for a time-out. I had to get up and press play again, and meanwhile I could ask him what the hell he was doing. I was a bit freaked.

"Do whatever you want to me," he said, legs and arms splayed across my bed.

I had no idea what to do.

"What are you doing? Do you do this with everyone?" I said.

He chuckled and said that the idea of my book was saturating our relationship. He'd been keeping dream journals for years and wanted to bring some of his own interests into the mix, hence the sleeping mask. Future-speak was in that sentence; it sounded to me like he was planning on sticking around for a while. I thought it was intoxicatingly sweet and managed quite well to show him how uncomplicated he was. The mask came off; his face contorted into a raisin and puffed back out into a grape again. My faculties remained intact as his collapsed into a blissful realm. I felt powerful while watching him buckle and warp. He opened his eyes and I stared into his left eye; it was a technique I had read in Barbara Carrellas's book, *Urban Tantra*. The left eye, it said, was the gateway to the soul. I wanted to see if I could connect Joe's soul to mine. But as I gazed, his eyes closed again and he convulsed into a depleted lump of contented flesh.

I felt like I was watching us from the cciling and couldn't believe the things I didn't know about this naked guy. I didn't know if he could use chopsticks. I didn't know if he left the toilet seat down. I didn't even know his favorite color. But I knew what he tasted like in my mouth.

He aimed to return the favor and shimmied down my body to show me, but I wasn't ready to unleash Clitty Rose's bouquet. Any guy who has ever tried to go down there gets caught in the scissors. My legs, like snakes, intertwine around them so they can't move closer to my juncture. I've always worried about the smell, the taste, and the look. I don't want a poor chap to be scarred. When I tell girlfriends I haven't had oral sex, they nearly always choke. Sometimes, if I bring it up with Fiona, I'm afraid she'll actually have a heart attack. So I squirmed around Joe until my legs were twisted tight. Unless he had a crowbar, he wasn't going to be able to unlock them. We cuddled and kissed and then lay still, my ass clicking perfectly into his fetal-positioned groin.

I pressed play on the CD again; I didn't want silence. He asked how many times I could listen to the same CD, as if repeat-mode was sacrilegious. He dressed and left the mask on my nightstand. He wanted me to test out my dreams with it, but it felt like he was leaving behind a piece of him to sleep with me. I walked him to the door. Our lips touched, and he left with a grin as loud as the creaking stairs. I went to the kitchen and had some ice cream—my culinary orgasm of the evening. I became self-conscious about my body developing a mint-chocolate-chip roll around my midsection. I stopped scooping. I went to the bedroom and took the sleeping mask to my nose and sniffed; it smelled thick and tired, like a room hot-boxed by marathon sleepers. I fell asleep with it in my hand and dreamed of kissing strangers.

During the next few days, some really sick stuff happened in my head. Embarrassingly sick. It nauseated me to know that I could think like this. See, I didn't want to settle down. I didn't want to depend on anyone. I didn't even know if I wanted a boyfriend. So when I saw fathers walking around my neighborhood with small cradled creatures at their chests and thought Joe would be cute with one of those multicolored slings attached to his shoulders, not only was I confused, but I also wanted to throw up. These thoughts couldn't be of my own volition. I blamed them on watching too many fabric-softener commercials where the mother figure somehow becomes brilliantly happy simply by rubbing her face all over her ruddy-complexioned kids' freshly washed underwear.

I was somehow forgetting that I wanted to be alone . . . but then again, I've seen people when they get older, when they are older and alone. No spouse, no kids, and they end up having perplexing bonds with their pets, practically frenching them in the park and cooing lovingly when they shit on the street. I didn't want to depend on anyone, but I didn't want to be a spinster either, lonely and cooking elaborate five-course meals for my lizards. (If you didn't notice, I'm not a mammal person. I have enough hair in my life already, and always in the wrong places.)

"Don't write him right away," said Leigh. "Don't call him, don't be too available."

But as sick as it made me, I kind of wanted to.

WINDOWS

Fiona's tour was in Connecticut. She rented a car to come into the city for the evening. When I hugged her, I felt the swivel of her interlocking vertebrae. She was skinnier than she'd ever been. She said she and Pedro were having problems.

I wished I didn't eat when I was in turmoil. I was feeling fatter than ever and there was another five-hundred-calorie bottle of wine yet to be uncorked. I tried to quell Fiona's anxieties as she quelled mine. "Mara, you're not fat," she said. Her quelling didn't work, so I asked her to tell me again. "Mara, you're not fat," she repeated. Damn it, it still didn't work, but it wouldn't be right to ask a third time, at least not as the precursors to tears began to accessorize her face—shiny eyes, tightened eyebrows, flushed cheeks, quivery nostrils. I tried to make them go away by making her laugh.

"Shut up," she said, half-laughing, her eyes still dewy. "I'm in distress, remember?"

We climbed onto my fire escape—the same one where Joe and I had most recently made out—and drank a bottle and a half of wine, getting louder while our livers tried to catch up with our consumption. We talked about regret, and about orgasms.

Fiona said sex was talking without talking. In a healthy relationship, she said, thrusting was a whole conversation. She used physical movement, friction, and sensation as a barometer in her love affairs. "I've been having orgasms since I was eleven," she said. "Now I want the ones that reverberate in my soul."

How can you get all picky about the type? I was thinking. *At least you have them!* But it felt like a bad time to say that.

"We're not making love," she said of Pedro. "We're just fucking. It's just sex."

I asked her if she had pussy nausea. It's a bad sign when you have pussy nausea. Pussy nausea is when you let something up there, usually of the male membranous type, and then when you think about it later, you have little pussy pangs of regret. I'd had it before.

"No," she said. "This time I have intuition nausea."

She'd followed her intuition when she got married after knowing Pedro for only two months, and now the marriage was unraveling before her eyes. For the past year and a half she'd been shocked every time she looked in the mirror. "I'm a wife!" she'd say to herself, unable to believe it.

"Maybe I wasn't meant to be married," she said. "I don't want to have kids. I don't want to buy a house with him. I don't want anything permanent."

She thought marriage would make everything come together. But for her, marriage set impossible parameters; it was like trying to cage an elephant with a cat carrier. She had grown up with my parents as an example as much as I had and thought that certified interdependency—becoming Fiondro or Peona—was the way to stem her insatiable urge for novelty. Being married, by law, meant till death do us part. She could focus on those words, instead of the next interesting guy to turn the corner. But it wasn't working.

As we dangled our feet out the window, she said she felt her decision surfacing. She didn't have to depend on Pedro for anything. "I don't even feel beautiful when he looks at me anymore," she said. "I want him to look into my eyes and know everything about me."

I reminded her that they'd been apart for four months while she was on tour. "Maybe that's part of it," I said.

"You're my best friend," she said. "You can't defend him!"

I didn't want to upset my best friend. I didn't want her to see my skepticism. But she knew me too well.

"Why are you looking at me like that?" she said.

Okay, I couldn't help rolling my eyes a little bit. She had a pattern. She was a serial girlfriend; she'd been someone's girlfriend since she was fifteen. I'd constantly lose her as she'd drown herself in the newness of an unknown personality. Each new boy she met was miraculously better than the last. She'd see all the characteristics that'd make him great—the opposite of me, since when I was looking, I could only concentrate on the traits that prevented a guy from being Mr. Right. "I've never felt this way before!" was her chorus line in any new relationship. I was always glad when she yodeled it over the phone rather than in person, so that I could roll my eyes in peace.

I guess I'm a little jealous of the way she could release and spontaneously dive openhearted into unknown possibilities. While she was busy falling in love and employing her flesh for orgasmic rewards, I was busy freaking out about things like death. I've been aware of sex and death for as long as I can remember; they seem like those things you just grow up knowing, like how to breathe, swallow, and release your bladder. But sex and death, which are supposed to be

one-size-fits-all notions, have never fit too well on me. I've been obsessed with death since I was seven, holding an anti-dying stance the
whole while. My parents don't believe in an afterlife, so my father's
way to console me was to tell me that I wouldn't know when I was
dead. I'd be six feet under. Black. Nothingness. It wouldn't matter at
all. The only good part about my subsequent freaking out was the
high I'd get from a lack of oxygen between my howls.

I'd think of how the globe looked from outer space, the green
continents floating in a sea of blue matter. I'd be buried somewhere
in craggy North America. There'd be a tombstone and a little tree
shading the grassy area. We plant evidence to show we existed.
We want to have a tombstone, to discover something, to win some
award, to write a book that might be remembered, to pass on our
genes, to make a ripple. A splash. An echo that's heard after our
bodies decay. But who remembers whatever we've left behind when
the world itself is gone?

An orgasm is a momentary detachment from life. The French
know it as *le petit mort*, the little death. Shakespeare wrote about
the connection between orgasm and death; the Tibetans did too.
Lose yourself in death, lose yourself in another person, lose yourself in life, let your senses flood. A detachment from conscious
thought, no space for logic; an eradication of identity; a loss of control. Orgasm is the essence of the thing to miss; it's life in concentrated form. It's even easier to feel like that's the case when you've
never had one, I guess.

"M," said Fiona. "It's an orgasm, a muscle spasm—not the end
of the world."

Wasn't it more, though? Orgasm had made Fiona second-guess
her marriage; it made me want to reexamine who I really was.

In the morning, Fiona and I went on a walk for coffee. We
watched toddlers scream, their faces pucker and turn into wrinkled

beets before bursting into fountains of salty water. Their owners exhaled.

The same questions continued to loom in Fiona's mind. If she got a divorce, would she regret it later? If she stayed, would she find herself at thirty-five with the need to start all over?

"I'm going to be a divorcée and I'm not even thirty," she said. "Didn't I get married for a reason? Wasn't there something I saw?"

People's perspectives are constructed from their own eyes, like customized windows on the world, but every window has smudges. We can clean or smudge our windows accordingly. Fiona wanted to see certain traits in Pedro at the beginning—wills are strong, especially hers—so those traits were formed, like his penchant for yoga and raw dehydrated banana-date loaves.

"Maybe marriage is an anachronistic institution," she said.

My windows agreed.

Before she left, I told her about Joe. I told her I felt weak when someone took over my thoughts like he did. I had a severe case of limerence. I'd smelled his sleeping mask so often that I thought I might have inhaled it all and now effused sleeping boy.

"Just ride the wave," Fiona said. "Trust yourself. Everything will be fine."

She took her own advice and took off, back to Connecticut, with clarity.

SOMETIMES I HATE MY BRAIN

There's a small mound of cement just outside ACE Bar's doorway. It's cruel, I know, but sometimes I go there between delivering drinks, seeking out my own sick entertainment by watching the tumult of the mating game. The little lump always catches people off guard, especially after the fourth cocktail and even more especially for a woman who has enhanced her booty-licious gait with high heels. Ankles tweak while hands flail and gravity pulls on her bottom faster than she was prepared for, but the stumble is always accompanied with a smile because the pain won't be felt until tomorrow. She's had too many and is caught up in a speedlike rush of dopamine and norepinephrine unleashed by the presence of her crush, who's stabilizing her in his arms. The infatuation-inducing hormones make the couple numb to the outside world, numb to the fact that the bouncer and I are chuckling at them. But when he touches her skin, she's anything but anesthetized; the sensation shoots 156 mph to her gray matter. I kind of feel sorry for them. They're prey to their own chemicals,

which manipulate them like a puppeteer would a marionette, om-
nisciently synchronizing their movements: She'll cross her legs,
and then he'll cross his. He'll take a drink, and she'll be only a
second behind. Where's free will? After a hug, one not much longer than twenty seconds, a small burst of oxytocin, the same stuff
that gushes during orgasm, floods their brains, especially hers.
For the woman, now arching her back as she tosses her hair over
her shoulder with a coy grin behind her jacket collar, the neuro-
chemical surge relaxes the amygdala and the anterior cingulate
cortex (the former alerts the body to fear, the latter controls critical thinking), so she'll be much more likely to disregard any of
the shortcomings her new lover might have and allow the mating
dance to take its course, for breeding—the species must go on.
They'll wake up tomorrow morning, scorning the evening; it was
all one big elaborate charade put on by brain plumbing. She'll
wonder why he wouldn't make eye contact and forgot to leave his
number when he left; he'll already be out the door and patting
himself on the back for not having swallowed the bait. It wasn't
time to be hooked but time to be a gardener; he's got to hoe up
the whole backyard before the seeds are sown.

What can I say? I felt irritable. I was premenstrual. And I'd
had what turned out to be my last date with Joe the day before.
While I'd waited in my apartment, pacing for the man I thought
of as my lover to arrive, I finally took my mascot, Picchu the vulva
puppet, out and shoved my hand up her backside. I manipulated
the stuffed labia as astutely as the brain chemicals had those two
strangers. Picchu warned me about the Vulvalution as passion-
ately as Paul Revere had warned the people of Boston about the
Revolution: "You will be coming! You will be coming!" I was
excited. I quickly stuffed Picchu back in her pink silk drawstring
bag and ran down the stairs to meet Joe. We spent an hour listen-

ing to live Brazilian music at a nearby bar. He held my hand as we strolled back to my apartment and he divulged his current career preoccupations. People don't share that stuff with just anyone, do they?

Okay, here's where it all fell apart: A different CD was already in my stereo to demonstrate my broader musical appreciation. I pressed play. We immediately started to roll around on my mattress. He was naked before I could count to five alligators, and I was stripped of all apparel save for my best pair of Old Navy black mesh panties. We turned into a mass of intertwined epidermis. It would have been impossible to figure out where my limbs ended and his began if it weren't for his black body hair to help distinguish. He whispered that he liked me and thought I was beautiful. All good signs, right? He dry-humped me practically to desiccation before we started to wonder if there was a condom. I could figure out that foreplay stuff later—later will always be the right time. We'd been on five dates. It was appropriate. I think. I thought. Whatever. We looked everywhere for a little aluminum packet.

He was straddling my belly, desperately digging into the recesses of his wallet. His scrotum dipped into my navel. Then thoughts came at me like sparrows at a window, relentless. The synergy between crotch and brain broke; I had questions. Aren't people supposed to be totally and utterly lost to reason while in the throes of passion? Damn it! Why was I thinking? I asked him if he'd been tested lately. He said yes, that he was clean. Then I said I had to know someone was really into me before I had sex with him. If ever a jaw went agape, his did.

The game exploded right there. We blew past the line and launched into uncharted Tempur-Pedic mattress territories. He asked if I was serious.

"Yes."

"I'm naked," he said, continuing to knock his wallet around.

He said he liked me and that he wanted to fuck me and he was sure he'd like to do it again and again, but that he wasn't ready for monogamy. He had just been in a relationship six months ago and wanted to see many women. I guess I had to give him points for honesty.

"I don't have an overwhelming urge to be in a relationship with you," he said.

Ouch: overwhelming urge. Did he have to put it that way? He wanted to know if I would date more. I said no. The game dies once you have an answer, and we were grounded in a refreshing haywire.

I got out from under him and switched the CD back to the one that I had played over and over on the date before. I felt liberated and free. I felt like me again. What had I let happen to me? In a fleeting moment of humor, he asked if we were entitled to breakup sex. I actually contemplated it; I wondered if that's what I needed. Maybe an orgasm would finally brew if there was nothing to lose. Ride the wave? But with my hesitation came foresight, and I knew the next day I'd have a void between my thighs and an irrepressible urge to download more of his MySpace songs. We cuddled while I told him that he was missing out. I told him that I was someone special; mostly, though, I was trying to convince myself. I mourned what I saw as my potential mate and orgasm coconspirator while he came to grips with the fact that I wouldn't be showing him how uncomplicated he was again. We both lamented the fact that we fit so well together and wouldn't discover if the last link really clicked.

He wouldn't take the sleeping mask back. I didn't want it . . . but I did. He left it by my bedside. I'm not going to fawn over hits of your musty, malodorous sleep vibes anymore! He asked if we could hang out as friends; of course I wanted to *not* as friends, but I kept silent and gave him this wistful, edgy look that I was hoping said something like, "Go suck your own cock!"

Then I went *fuck fuck fuck* all the way to the fridge.

I WOULD HEREBY LIKE TO SUE
MYSELF FOR DEFAMATION

"You're intellectualizing, Mara," said Rori. I was in her office again. Even though the appointment was once a week, I felt like I was perpetually there. Here I am where I am again.

"But what do you feel?" she continued. "You said Joe didn't want to be in a relationship with you and that's fine with you?"

I smiled. It hurt to smile. I'd chewed a cheek lump the size of an erect nipple. "Yeah, I'm fine," I said. "I don't want one anyway. It's just a waste of time."

"That doesn't mean it doesn't hurt," she said.

I wasn't going to cry for something I didn't believe in. It was just the nice smile coupled with a penis that confused me. Joe had been a momentary bout of insanity.

Breakups were in the air. Across the country, Fiona was prepping Pedro for divorce. She was already reading *Eat, Pray, Love* by Elizabeth Gilbert. She had heard from her mother, who had heard from Oprah, that it was a must-read for every soon-to-be divorcée. She said she was going to go on a self-finding mission in an Indian ashram as soon as her tour was up in February. "I'm just going to meditate," she said. "I'm going to find myself." I didn't say anything. Who was I to say where "herself" would or wouldn't turn up?

About a week later, I received a package from Joe. I giggled all the way upstairs and took my time opening it, thinking maybe it was an apology, a jack-in-the-box that when wound up would jump out and say, "Oops, I meant to say I *do* have an overwhelming urge to be with you!" But no, there were six sex books inside: *The Female Brain*, *Sperm Counts*, *A History of Sin*, *Impotence*, and *The Humble Little Condom* (maybe he should have kept that as a reminder to himself for later on). A small yellow Post-It note was stuck on the last one, hiding its title: *Virgin*.

The note said, "Mara—thought these might help with research—Joe."

My roommates tried to comfort me, saying it was a convoluted way to say he wanted me. But I felt like he was taunting me, an I-know-how-to-orgasm-and-you-don't kind of thing. I propped them against the wall. They became a stool. I rubbed my ass on them.

As if I wasn't feeling sufficiently lame enough at that point, one of my five and a half called around this time to tell me someone had sent him an Internet link: "Mara Altman Is Writing a Book About How She Has Never Orgasmed." He said he was sorry that people were posting such mean things about me, and he was sure if I contacted the Webmaster, the erroneous post could be taken down.

I had to give him one of these: Well, um, actually . . .

He already knew I'd never had an orgasm. I'd told him that before; but he didn't know about my attempt to write a book about it and obviously couldn't believe it. To say the least, he wasn't pleased. He became defensive. It seemed that he felt *my* lack of orgasm all of a sudden had somehow wronged *him*, as if my talking about anorgasmia would reflect poorly upon his manhood because I'd been with him. I'd sullied him, and he didn't want the world to know about it.

"But it wasn't you," I said, trying to quell him. "It was me."

I don't know if I sounded convincing, but I believed what I was saying. Even though I'd spent all those years waiting for a guy to make me come, I didn't blame the ones who couldn't. I'd hardly made it easy for them.

He hung up less than pleased. Were the two—his good name and my anorgasmia—so closely intertwined that I was defaming him? If anyone, wasn't I defaming *myself*?

It reminded me of a miscommunication I'd had with a French man at ACE Bar, which had led to an enlightening conversation.

Me: You want some beers?

Man: What? You want to know my fears?

Me: Okay, what are your fears?

Man: My biggest fear is that I don't satisfy a woman.

Me: Why?

Man: Because then I've failed.

Me: Failed what?

Man: Failed to be a good lover.

Me: What if she fakes it?

Man: That'd be worse.

Me: Why?

Man: Because she would be doing it just to please me.

Me: At least your ego would be spared.

Man: It's not my ego.

Me: Then what is it?

Man: It's my fear.

It seemed that men were almost hijacking female pleasure to bolster themselves. I decided to reach out to people on Craigslist personals to find the relationship between the male psyche and the female orgasm. I figured there were many people there who'd collected some knowledge of the subject along their way to becoming professional Internet sex prowlers. I ended up meeting a few of them and interviewing them at Bleecker Bar.

Many confirmed what I had guessed: they said that they defined their sexual success in terms of how many times and how fast they could make a girl come. "When she gets there, it's like climbing the mountaintop," said Andrew, a thirty-eight-year-old who said he only uses Craigslist when he and his girlfriend are having trouble. "It's great to get laid, but once you make her come and put her to bed, you feel like a man." Another man wouldn't stop talking about how he was done with the female orgasm. "I've been so worried about her orgasm," he said, "that I'm the one who has trouble letting go." I also found that these men tend to prefer women who know what they want and are not afraid to express it. I figured that was because they sensed that if the girl knew about her own body, they would have a lower orgasm-failure rate. "Oh, men like freaky bitches," a twenty-eight-year-old man said. "Most dudes like a freak, a girl who's down and dirty. A chick who screams out what she likes." One guy even told me that making his girlfriend come inspires creativity; he told me about different fish recipes he'd dreamed up during her climax, such as his roasted filet of halibut marinated in tabbouleh salad and a half-cup of lemon juice.

After all my interviews, I felt that orgasm might have been thrown into the mix just to stymie male-female relationships. I didn't know how I'd even managed two-month couplings without coming; men seemed so dependent on them. But even though I'd expected my first orgasm to come from a man, I was kind of pissed they were impinging on its ownership. It was mine! Well, wasn't it?

I WOULD HEREBY LIKE TO SUE MYSELF FOR DEFAMATION

I went to Atman, at the muffin stall, to talk it over. Ever since my last visit, I'd come to think of him as my crotch guru.

He stood by a mountain of bulk apples. His eyes darted toward me. He touched my forehead and kissed both cheeks.

"Oh, sweetie," he said, grabbing my hands and kissing them. "It's a lovely day. You've come for more about your flower?"

"Yes, my flower," I said, relenting. If it was anything botanical, Clitty Rose was more of a humid greenhouse, but I didn't say so.

I tried to direct the discussion, but he wouldn't have any of my talk about egos, male or otherwise. He wasn't into ego. He started his own strain of conversation.

"You need tolerance and patience," he said. "Start running before crawl, we get hurt."

Then he started telling me about the karma points I'd accrued from past lives in Europe and Scandinavia. I wondered why Atman could look into the past but not let me in on some quick orgasmic fix. He obviously didn't understand deadlines.

"We are more natural and fruitful than fictional," he said. "Cleanse your alchemy. Eat seasonal fruit and seasonal vegetation; not from storage coming from California and Florida—no, coming from local."

"And that will help me with my flower?" I said. I was staring at a zucchini the size of Betty's gigantic black dildo, the Nimbus.

"Not so ambitious," he said. "Neutral, not judgmental or opiniative. Be with your curiosity."

Curiosity. My mind went immediately to the Jersey City dungeon, which I'd almost forgotten about. Barry, the BDSM guy, didn't seem like he needed his ego stroked. He got enough of whatever it was he was after with his fisting routines. Atman kissed me between my eyebrows as people waved their dollar bills in exchange for his goodies. I walked away, rifling through my wallet for the little slip that read MASTERS OF PAIN.

NOAH'S ARK

I left a phone number and address for Leigh and Ursula before I took the PATH train to Jersey City.

Barry picked me up at the station. I entered the Masters of Pain headquarters, a somewhat dilapidated three-story home. I put on my best nonpartisan reporter face, but I was glad no one was paying attention to me as I scanned the walls, as I could feel my face contorting in all manners of judgment.

Framed photos of women in compromising positions were scattered randomly around his brick-wall living room. Stills of girls dressed in black crying tears of blood, their mouths covered with duct tape with "slut" written on it, gaped at me. Knee-length patent leather boots were collapsed onto themselves in the corner. The TV was blaring with no one watching. On the table, there were fifty DVD cases waiting to be packed. The cover photo was of a naked young woman, her nipples clamped and pulled forward, her labia twisted and elongated by dangling forceps. Her face, crumpled in pain, was the same color of red as the ambiguous tattoo humping her waistline. The title was *The Torture of Sunshine*.

"Sunshine," yelled Barry. "Sunshine!"

A young woman with jeans and a T-shirt galloped down the stairs. Her hair was in a haphazard ponytail. She was younger than his son, Bam Bam, and had a ball-bearing piercing where Marilyn Monroe's iconic mole sat.

"I need you to pack these," ordered Barry, pointing to the discs. "We're taking them into the city tomorrow."

"Can I have lunch money," she whined. "I'm hungry."

She gave me an out-of-the-corner-of-her-eye look of contempt. I was staring at her heavily tampered-with majora on the package and couldn't fathom she'd be pleased I knew so much about her, while all she knew of me was that I carried around blue Bic writing utensils. Barry pulled out a twenty and put it into her palm. Her poor vulva—I wondered if it'd reclaimed its shape by now. She traipsed into the sunlight as Barry took me down to the dungeon for a tour. He wore a sky blue T-shirt that too closely matched his acid-wash jeans and Reebok tennis shoes, which in their just-out-of-the-box whiteness contrasted disturbingly with the floor's off-white carpeting below their soles. There were no bars or cells down there, just the mustiness of a basement that's been chewing on its own debris for too long. There were hospital gurneys and a whole slew of tools lined up along the wall. There were handcuffs, St. Andrew's crosses, whips, dildos of every size attached to elaborate strap-on halters, knives, and bench press equipment. There was a box whose contents I was trying to discern. Barry helped me out.

"Oh, that's an enema kit," he said. "One of the girls gave one to a guy in the last film."

"Interesting," I said, mentally patting myself on the back for my casual air.

Barry switched off the light before I had had a good look around, but I didn't protest. He didn't give me a moment to question his control. I followed him up two flights of stairs. He entered his bedroom. I followed. He sat in front of his computer. There was no other chair, just an unmade bed and another elaborate collection of toys hooked along the wall.

"I don't play in the dungeon," he said. "I do all my playing in here."

He said he had had a woman over the night before. He had taken two of his vibrators to her and made her come five times.

"That's what I do," said Barry. "I'm here to help people out. I give away what I got for free."

I practiced nonjudgment, but I sure as hell was not about to sit on his playground. The sheets were helter-skelter, as though sharks had been thrashing in them.

He started clicking on the mouse and said he had to place an ad on Craigslist for Sunshine.

I'm 5'10" and 135 pounds with dark hair. I do both types of role play, foot worship, cbt, strap on, feminization, humiliation and more. I'm a dom not an escort. This is strictly about domination.

Sunshine was a professional dominatrix; Barry's dungeon was her office. She put unfulfilled spouses and boyfriends in women's panties, whipped them, and gave them enemas for two hundred dollars an hour; Barry kept half as commission. He lived well off a never-ending supply of sexually unfulfilled men.

I was still standing.

"Go grab a chair from downstairs," he said, "and tell Sunshine to get a cup of water."

"I don't need water," I said, trying to be an easy and gracious guest.

"No," he said. "*I* want water."

"Oh," I said, befuddled. I went downstairs. Sunshine was pouring milk over a bowl of Apple Jacks.

"Barry wants water," I said.

"The cups are there," she said, pointing to a drying rack full of plastic White Castle cups and not even looking at me. I filled up the cup.

Barry took the cup from my hands without a word—not even a thank you—and began explaining domination and submission. I stared at the diamond earring in his left ear and his elongated widow's peak, from which all other hair receded like water around a sand bar.

"Are you hetero, homosexual, bi, bi-curious?"

"Uh, I guess I'm heterosexual-very-timid," I said.

"Oh, so you need someone to take control," he said. "See, most women are submissive, but what happens is they grow up being submissive but unappreciated. You need someone who's dominant and willing to explore your heart and then your body. If I build you up to be the best submissive you can be for me, then you're going to be pleasing me, which will have rewards that will be pleasing to you, if I train you properly."

Some people play dom/sub as a sex game. Barry lived it.

He went on to explain that he had three rules for his submissives. He said it all as matter-of-factly as an accountant would discuss tax code. They must always be naked when inside his house, always fill his water, and always ask permission to use the bathroom and keep the door open when they do.

"Like kids, submissives are going to test to see if they can get away with things," he said. "In order for you to respect me, I'm going to have to confront that situation when it happens."

One of his subs once forgot to fill his water cup; he made her carry around a full cup of water for twenty-four hours so she would remember next time. He said if I forgot to ask for permission to use the bathroom, he'd make me shit in diapers.

I kept listening, but I really hoped he'd stop saying "you."

"You know the bottom line," he said. "I cherish you, I love you, I protect you, and that's all someone wants from their lover. Honesty and trust."

Was he auditioning me?

I checked out a movie poster pinned to his bulletin board. It pictured Barry sitting in a chair with a blond-headed girl bent over one knee. A g-string over red-splotched buttocks was just below his swinging palm. "The Punishment of Crista," it read, "starring Sir B with Little C." Sir B was Barry's stage name.

He said the sub got off on the endorphins that came from pleasing the dom, while the dom got off on having control.

"My trip comes from the fact that you trust me enough to give me your body to do these things to you," he said. "That's my power trip. Sometimes I'm so focused on what I'm doing that there's no time for the arousal to hit my cock, no hard-on. That's a trip."

I continued staring at the shiny diamond in his ear and let him ramble on. He asked me questions, but not many answers came to mind. Screw endorphins, I thought. Who actually needs endorphins? I can take a jog for endorphins.

"You need to be in a relationship with me or someone just like me for at least the next six months to a year," he said. "Somebody—and I'm not talking about a committed-committed relationship—who can be there with you and take you through all these things you need to explore and understand."

I really needed to be home all of a sudden.

I told him maybe it wasn't my thing.

NOAH'S ARK

"Remember, orgasms aren't about love. They are about pleasure. You don't have to be in love with someone," he said. "An orgasm is not a thing of intimacy; it's a fucking thing of pleasure. It's like eating an ice cream cone. If you like chocolate, you go to the store and buy chocolate. See what I'm saying?"

Sir B was finally starting to make a little sense. Orgasm was a muscle reflex, a sensation. He was right! I'd taken the wrong path, like I had my whole life, when I went for Joe. I didn't need Joe or emotions to figure this thing out. Sir B naturally separated love, intimacy, and sex like oil and water. My problem was that I'd gotten them all intertwined. I needed to unbraid them.

"If someone said, 'Here's one hundred million dollars, but you can never have orgasms or sex again,' would you take it? Fuck no! Fucking life is all about pleasure. Don't deny yourself anything; life is too short. This is what it's about. Get your priorities straight!"

I could tell he was trying to rattle me out of my timidity. He could be construed as pervy, but I think he genuinely wanted me to discover what he saw as the biggest treasure all people have locked inside: the pleasure of their sexuality.

"Pleasure," I said, rolling it around on my tongue.

I swallowed that word while he got up to plug in his double-headed Magic Wand vibrator.

"What are you doing?" I asked.

"This is what I used last night," he said, holding the machine as it pulsated. "Five orgasms. Come on, touch it."

"I better go now," I said.

"I washed it," he said. "Just touch it."

These sex people, why do they always want you to touch stuff that's been inside other people? I stretched out my pinkie and touched it fast, like it was hot.

Then he told me about the foot fetish party he had scheduled at Paddles, the only S&M club in New York City, for the following week. He told me I should come, that it'd be interesting for research. We went downstairs. Sunshine and Pixie, another dominatrix, were slumped on the sofa watching the *Tyra Banks Show* and perusing their MySpace pages, waiting for their next clients to show. Sir B took me to the train station.

He said I should do exercises at home. I should lie in bed, close my eyes, breathe, and touch myself.

"Take your hands and let them go," he said. "Let your mind go wherever. If your mind goes to a place where you're being fucked by a horse, let it go. It's okay; let it go. Go with it. Don't stop, just touch yourself."

I got out of the car, holding my tainted pinkie finger outstretched and away from my body. At least I'd indulged my curiosity; Atman would be proud of me. Sir B reminded me once more about my homework assignment.

"Think of me in the corner of your room," he said. "I'm smiling and approving of every movement that you make. I'm just smiling at you and nodding and saying, 'Yes, good, very good.'" As if he were in my room already, he nodded his head, grinning.

That night I got into bed. I pulled up my shirt and started touching my stomach. I felt the slight rise of my belly and the undulations of my rib cage. As I got closer to my groin, Sir B appeared in the corner; he was smiling and coaxing me to go further. Then the horse Sir B had mentioned appeared. It had one of those creepy raw-hot-dog-looking horse schlongs. Then more animals—cheetahs, elephants, giraffes—arrived, and even Sir B's dominatrix chicks came aboard. Within two minutes, I'd managed to re-create Noah's ark in my room. There was hardly any room for me on the bed. My body tensed up. I couldn't touch myself in front of all of them. After all, they weren't the ones I was trying to please.

NOAH'S ARK

FOOTNOTES

"I went to a foot fetish party last Saturday night," I said, riffing on a moment that'd been playing over and over in my head for three days and four nights.

Rori calmly crossed her legs. She customarily wears no jewelry, no wedding ring, no indicators beyond the Diet Peach Snapples she drinks to construct what her life is like beyond this office building, but I guess at it anyway. I bet she has orgasms. She looks like she has a lot of orgasms.

She nodded, bangs falling forward. "Yeah, continue."

I told her that someone had sucked my foot, practically had sex with it. He paid me one hundred dollars for fifty minutes. I said I was conflicted.

"Why?"

I liked it.

I hadn't gone to the party to be a participant. If someone had asked me prior to it if I'd prefer to get my toes sucked by a stranger or weed the thousands of plants in my parents' nursery,

I would have selected the latter. I went because Sir B thought it'd be good for me; he didn't let the fact that I had declined his first propositions—using his double-headed Magic Wand or getting naked and shitting in his toilet with the door open—deter him. He suggested I come to the Paddles Club in Chelsea to observe how the BDSM world worked; he wanted to break down my inhibitions.

I went right after work; I was in jeans and a T-shirt and had on the little green and gold flats I've worn pretty much every day for the last year and a half. When I find a comfortable pair, I wear them until they disintegrate. I wouldn't wish their stench—which was odoriferously related to a burnt batch of my father's famous cheddar cheese–snapper flambé decomposing in a Dumpster for a week—upon anyone.

After descending into a basement, I was confronted with a big, brightly painted mural. In it, a cartoonish woman in bright purple spandex leaned against an enormous penis, which shot out from moon-crater-looking land. One of her high heels stabbed the cock's shaft; a metal bar pierced its head. Another woman had a man on a skin-pinching leash, while he stuck his gas-masked head into a bin of green toxic waste.

Against that backdrop, women in three-inch platforms picked at potato chips and popcorn in heart-embossed bowls. Sodas and juices were served in Dixie cups. The club didn't own a liquor license, so attendees would run to the bar across the street to throw one back and quickly return. The ladies each looked like half-packed sausages: their corsets and mini dresses only cased their midsections; buttocks and breasts were left bulging out at each end. Meanwhile, I hid behind my multiple hemlines.

Sir B made purposeful steps toward me; the breeze from the forward motion ruffled his hair, making a tidal wave over his sand bar.

He had too much conviction for it to be a good sign. He grabbed my arm.

"Mara, I've got a customer for you," he said. "He wanted a little girl; you're the littlest one I've got."

"What?" I didn't mean to come off as dumb, but it was my version of the ostrich's life-saving technique: sticking its head in the sand.

I said absolutely not. I hadn't come to work the party. First Sir B wanted me to be his submissive slave; now he was a gigolo for my extremities? Look at the other girls' feet, all strappy, glossily polished, and porcelain-colored. Those were the feet to get busy with. My feet were ugly; they were wide, smelly, and dirty, with chipped nail polish and a mutant pinkie toenail.

"Barry, listen to me," I said. "I've had bunion surgery. Bunions! That's the most anti-sexy surgery in the world."

Sir B took my elbow. "Some guys like that shit," he said, dragging me toward a middle-aged man with a head of white hair in a blue polo. He sat in the corner of a maroon sofa.

"Take your shoes off," Sir B ordered as I looked up at him. "Come on," he said, narrowing his brow. "Just take them off. It's not gonna kill you."

I slipped off my disintegrating flats.

The guy, whose name was Fred, assessed my right foot. He held it for a second. "They're gross," I said, praying the poor man wouldn't breathe in through his nose. Sir B scowled at me and put a finger over his lips. "Shush!"

The guy gave one last appraisal, with a pinch. "They're great," he said. "Beautiful."

I smiled. This crazy fetishist dude liked my ugly feet. Sir B sent me off to the restroom with a towel and a bottle of witch hazel to clean them up. Was I delusional? I started laughing at my reflection in the bathroom mirror. I tried to balance with one foot in the sink as a woman in a skintight nurse's uniform entered.

"Hey, how are you supposed to react when someone's playing with your feet?" I asked.

"You let them lick them or whatever," she said, re-jiggering her breasts. "Pretend you like it. Say, 'Oh, that feels so good,' and then breathe a little heavy."

"My feet are so ugly, though," I said, showing her, hoping she'd counter my opinion. She just shrugged her shoulders, turned, slammed the stall door, and started peeing.

Sir B grabbed me as I exited and brought me back to the sofa. I sat on the opposite end from Fred. He slipped forty dollars into my palm. It was hard to take the money. Did pocketing it make me a whore? Fred placed the soles of my feet on his chest. He began stroking them. He closed his eyes. Other people were watching. We were on display in the middle of the club. Strangers walked by in rubber suits, buckles fastened around their wrists and ankles, clanking with each step. Sir B was to the right of me, whipping a girl who was up against the wall like da Vinci's Vitruvian Man.

Fred brought my right foot to his mouth and starting kissing it softly. He treated each toe pad like it was a mouth and made out with it. His favorite was the pad just below my big toe; he sucked on it, and took a nibble. He caressed my calf and Achilles tendon like one might the head and neck during a normal make-out session; the ankles were the ears and he fondled them. Fred gave me twenty dollars more and then another forty. He wanted the session to last longer. I gazed up at the ceiling and realized I'd never loved my feet as much as I did with this stranger nuzzling them. The money did something quite opposite from what I had thought possible: it was liberating.

FOOTNOTES

"What you're saying," said Rori, "is that you felt liberated when he objectified you?"

Yeah, I guess so. The transaction was clear: he gave me money and I gave him access to my feet. There was no "What next?" in the equation. I didn't have to worry about falling in love or about his intentions post–timer beep. Fred split me into parts, but I felt more whole than ever. I was finally in the moment. I even let out a pleasure-induced *mmm* just remembering it.

"I don't get it," I said to Rori. "How was I okay with that, but I can't manage to be in the moment with anyone I potentially have the capability of actually liking?"

I fidgeted with her sofa pillows and slammed my back into the cushions.

"You know, I don't actually want to be 'one' with someone," I said. "It's only society that ever made me think I did."

"But Mara, society is real," she said. "Those feelings it creates are a fact of life. Ignoring those feelings is only rationalizing them through logic, and feelings are not a logical thing."

·But how real could feelings be? I'd just found out my feelings were swayed by mere symmetry. I'd begrudgingly cracked open *The Female Brain*, one of the books Joe had sent me. I read that women are more attracted to symmetrical men. We don't even really know we're doing it; it's subconscious, ruled by some Stone Age remnant of the brain. We want to have symmetrical men's babies because their sperm are supposedly hardier little suckers. Symmetricals have it made; statistically, the book said, they spend less money and time on their dates but still have intercourse sooner than their cockeyed counterparts.

"I looked at Joe's picture after I read that," I said. "Guess what, he's symmetrical. Evan was, too. I fell victim to some ancient genetic mind trap. I didn't like them, my genes did."

"So now you're not going to take responsibility for who you are, for what you like?" she said. "You're going to credit heredity and hormones for all of your emotions?"

She looked at me from the corner of her eye, one of those looks that said, You see it now, don't you?

"Maybe I'm just agitated because I'm PMS-ing," I said.

Even if my period had just ended, I'd always tended to blame my bad moods on PMS—because, really, a female is premenstrual until she's menstrual, at which point she can transfer the blame of her irritation to it being "that time of the month." But then for the first time, I realized what I'd said: I had given my uterus the right, just like I had my Stone Age brain, to determine who I was again. Rori didn't have to pat herself on the back; I could see it in her eyes.

"Where is the *you* in all these experiences?" she said. "You're in there somewhere."

The *me* inside me was saying the best thing to do, in order to get my orgasm, was to separate love and orgasm, like what Sir B had said in his dungeon. One was emotional; the other was a physical reaction—so different, but so linked in my mind. When they were together, they always led to hurt and distraction.

I'd called myself a prude, but Fred had just paid me to use my body. I let him. I liked it. That's not very prudish. Maybe I had preemptively defined myself as a prude and tried to live by it all these years to make sense to myself. Because what do you do when you're not the type you thought you were anymore? You have to find out what else you might be.

Enough with the old Mara mythologies: it was time to embrace other possibilities.

THE GASM

OneTaste. OneTaste. OneTaste. I'd been hearing about OneTaste, a group of beings who supposedly lived orgasmically. The idea behind it, or what I'd heard of it, had initially creeped me out. I had heard they specialized in the female orgasm and doing a thing called OMing—Orgasmic Meditation—where they put all attention on the genitals and, through that, became enlightened. Or something like that. This idea wasn't allowed to creep me out anymore because I'd just decided I was no longer a prude, and now it was time to prove it. If all I heard was true and they really did know so much about the female orgasm, and even lived for the orgasm, maybe they'd even know the MEANING OF ORGASM. Not to put it in capital letters or anything.

The walls were all white. The flooring in their Chinatown base was made of polished wood. People gathered in a circle for their weekly meeting called In Group. The leader, Racheli Cherwitz, greeted me.

"Do you know how, in yoga, people focus on the breath?" she asked.

I nodded.

"Well, here, we focus on the orgasm."

Racheli was twenty-six years old and so slender she could slip through a full row at the movie theater without anyone having to stand up. She had brown, closely cropped hair. Her gaze was a less deranged and more feminine version of Marshall Applewhite's from that Heaven's Gate cult from the nineties, but just as severe. I felt like she was using her eyes like surgical lasers, deconstructing me as I sat in the chair opposite her.

"What happens with sex is there is all this other stuff left on top—love, relationship, family, kids—and it gets a little bit muddled," Racheli said. "I've had times in my life when I had a hot make-out with a guy and we ended up in a relationship and I didn't know why. We just had a hot make-out, which was it. So what we're doing essentially is decoupling or separating the actual sensation in the body from the story behind it."

That's exactly what I was looking for.

Then she began explaining the practice.

"So what happens is, a woman lies down," Racheli explained. "She takes off her pants. The stroker, who can be male or female, will take his left index finger, put a dime of lubricant on the part of the pad where, if you got a paper cut, it would be most sensitive. He'll then stroke from the introitus [the entrance of the vaginal orifice] up and over to the left-hand quadrant of the clit. He'll take the thumb and put it in the introitus to lock down the energy. It closes the circuit. So then once he's on the upper left-hand quadrant, the ten o'clock spot, he'll stroke up, down, up, down with differing speeds for fifteen minutes."

Words like "circuit," "quadrant," "energy," and "lock down" made my new-age radar bleep. I didn't know if I trusted New Age speak, but I persevered and promised myself I wouldn't wake up the next day with a batch of sprouted raw almonds in my kitchen and Yanni playing on my stereo.

Racheli continued. She said they weren't the first group to use this method. It went back to a commune-type establishment called Lafayette Morehouse, previously known as More University, which was established by a man named Dr. Victor Baranco in 1968. Racheli said he learned the OMing practice, which has since been adapted and changed over time, from a woman called the Witch.

"Who's the Witch?"

"The Witch is the Witch," she said.

"Oh," I said, being agreeable.

From there, the practice branched out into different orgasm communities. She briefly told me about one small family who now had orgasms all day long somewhere out in the California woods. She said she'd heard they were a bit hermetic and quite private. Hearing that made me immediately intrigued; I wanted to meet them.

"Orgasm is the highest state of sensation that the body experiences," she continued. "People will touch their purpose in that state. It's the closest we get to touching creation."

She said their headquarters were in San Francisco, where the founder, Nicole Daedone, lived. Racheli said Daedone was unbelievably orgasmically savvy. By the tone of her voice when she said it, I wouldn't have been surprised if she had unfurled an air mattress at that moment, gotten on her knees, and prayed in the direction of San Francisco. I told Racheli about my project and that I'd like to have an interview with Ms. Daedone. She told me their leader was too busy, and I'd be better off checking out her YouTube clips on the OneTaste website.

There were about eighteen people at this meeting, which was a weekly get-together designed to explore our desires. This wasn't one where everyone took off her pants, apparently. Racheli said I could come and take my pants off during the OMing circles; it only cost $250 to be initiated into taking your pants off. I took my pants off for free at home, but I didn't say that because she had those intense eyes and probably knew it's what I was thinking anyway.

We only had to pay ten dollars to participate in this discussion. After the meeting, everyone mingled. I met a man named Forrest. He told me more about Ms. Daedone. She seemed like an underground hero, a gift from the divine, the empress of all things below the waistline. She could read minds; she could make someone cry by placing her hand on their chest. She sounded like a cult leader. How often do you find yourself in the middle of a sex cult? And Ms. Daedone seemed like the perfect one to tell me the MEANING OF ORGASM. She was the opposite of The Anti-Gasm; she was, obviously, The Gasm.

"Are you sure I couldn't get an interview with Nicole Daedone?" I asked Racheli again.

"I'll ask," she said, "but I suggest YouTube for now."

As I was about to slip out the door, I introduced myself to one woman who'd caught my attention during the meeting. She'd sat Indian-style in her metal folding chair. Her cheeks were flushed. She was smiling constantly. As she spoke, she thumped up and down. That must have been a part of living orgasmically.

She said her name was Zola. She said I reminded her of herself before her sexual opening. I asked if she'd meet me for coffee the following week. She agreed.

THE PUSSY POETESS DEMANDS AN APOLOGY

When I spotted Zola waiting for me at the coffee shop, I could tell she was going to be my sexual Socrates. She was the sexualized version of the me I was striving to be—me cloned and then coated with some erotic emulsion. I was the same height as Zola—same brown eyes and brown hair too—but her figure was more curvaceous, as if her abundance of sexual energy were pounding against all the right feminine locations—breasts, hips, belly, and behind. Her eyes were as bright as her skin was smooth. I swear that orgasms must get rid of acne and red eye better than a cocktail of Visine and Clearasil ever could.

Zola was a pussy princess. She worked with pussy. Her favorite body part was the pussy. In her twenty-nine years, she had acquired infinite pussy factoids: much of the clitoris structure is internal—it's actually more than seven inches long, shaped like a wishbone—and it has the most nerve endings, eight thousand, concentrated in one spot than any other part of the human body.

She told me she was currently working on some Taoist exercises.

She'd insert a jade egg into her vagina to build strength inside. She was currently working on rotating the egg in a figure eight—no hands—while in a deep state of meditation.

I tried to measure up. I told her I could jog 3.5 miles in forty minutes while listening to music—and sometimes even chewing gum at the same time.

She pinched off a piece of a muffin. She made a sound with every morsel she munched, as if it'd activated her G-spot. She'd close her eyes for a few seconds in afterglow and then come right back to the conversation. With Zola, it was as if an orgasm was never very far away.

Zola started as a devout Catholic, then became a butch lesbian, then moved to New York and gave happy endings. Now she's bisexual and a Tantra teacher, also called a *dakini*. She teaches breathing and sex techniques to those who hope to reach higher sexual potentials. For three hundred dollars an hour, eight hundred for three, she will be your nude therapist. She'll listen to your bisexual fantasies. She'll eye-gaze, reverse impotence, validate your penis size, and cheer you on as you cross-dress for the first time. She basically gives space for you to explore your sexuality. She'll also fuck you in the ass with a strap-on dildo, if that's your thing. She'd classify herself as a sex worker, but she doesn't have sexual intercourse with her clients. "I'm a spy in the temple of love," she said. "I love my life!"

And I could tell she loved it; she squealed when she swallowed the blueberry in the muffin. She moaned as her coffee went down.

I told her my most recent problem. I thought that being the pussy professional that she was, she would have a solution. The problem revealed itself in my last session with Rori. Rori said I talked about my brain and body as if they were two different beings; I compartmentalized them. Rori's arms were spread to dem-

THE PUSSY POETESS DEMANDS AN APOLOGY

onstrate. The right hand, she said, was my brain; the left was my crotch. "We want to unify," she had said, bringing her hands together until they were parallel. "Sex and the mind don't have to be mutually exclusive."

"I think my pussy is autistic," I told Zola.

Zola mulled.

"Court your pussy," she demanded. "Seduce the hell out of her, woo her, find out what turns her on and off, take photos of her, buy flowers and chocolate."

"My pussy can't eat chocolate," I said. I had horrendous visuals as I said that.

She took another bite of muffin, moaning as she masticated.

"Your pussy is you!" she finally managed to say after swallowing. "What your pussy wants, you want!"

I scrunched my nose.

"Write her poetry," she said. "And seriously, don't call *her* an 'it.' She's a *she*."

As we parted, Zola gave me some books and a DVD called *Divine Nectar*, which she described as "a must-see" and "so beautiful it almost puts a tear in your eye."

When I got home that night, I sat down to type.

Dear Pussy,

I'm sorry that we've been out of touch. I want to get to know you. I want to know what makes you tick—or rather, what makes you twitch.

I know I haven't been the best pussy-keeper. I've kept you coddled and locked up in outdated underwear. I've abused my power—'cause let's face it, you're easily reigned over. While I can jump up and scream from excitement, you can only tingle and swell. I never splurge on the tampons with bleach-free cotton, and let's not even talk about the ninety-nine-cent one-ply I've used for wiping. If I get you waxed—which is uncommon these days, due to your lack of male interaction (I'll take the blame for that)—I take you to the cheapest places I can find, where you're destined to come out looking asymmetrical, with a plethora of ingrown hairs and a slight chance of being maimed. I realize that's not good for any girl's self-image—especially yours, as you're already ugly enough. No offense, we've discussed your looks before.

Okay, that was rude. I'm sorry. You're a flower. You're a conch. You're an iridescently fantastic orchid, a craggy mountain range, the awe-inspiring grandeur of a freshly cracked geode. Maybe I'm a little envious of the way men always seem to want you before me. But I should give you credit, you definitely have better instincts to deal with them. You get all beefed up and ready for interaction, while I get all defensive and say things I don't mean. Maybe I'd learn something by letting you take the lead.

But why did you go and develop your little magic button so far away from the point of penetration? In pussy mileage, the clit is about a marathon away. That's made undue hassle for me since before we lost our virginity. And the smell—come on, girl, did you have to develop a stink like that just to show people you were there?

I'm sorry. Sorry for the digression. This is to mend our differences. We've had fun times together. Remember the first time you queefed? I laughed so hard that you did it again just to please me. I guess what I'm really saying is that if we worked together—you know, developed a synergy—things could be better for the both of us. I'm going to try harder to listen to you. Maybe it will help once we start sleeping together. I'm going

THE PUSSY POETESS DEMANDS AN APOLOGY

to take Atman's advice on that. Last time I visited him, as I was about to walk away, mothers and small children gazing horrified, as always, in our direction, he called out, "Air ventilation! We tighten that part with so many layers. Stinky and smelly, you know, because the sweat, you don't let things get breath. Let the flower be free!"

So I'm going to let you be free. You deserved the fresh air long ago. I'm sorry, please forgive me. Let's start over as *one*, not me and you.

Love,
Mara

I began sleeping naked. I found myself waking up with my hand cupping my groin—there was a bond between the body parts I wasn't conscious existed. They acted as if they were long-lost lovers who'd been reunited. As I stared, the union would quickly break apart as teenagers do when caught dry-humping in public spaces.

I was feeling more adventurous than ever. I hadn't spoken to Betty, the Mother of Masturbation, for more than a month, but I even sent an e-mail to her young boyfriend, Eric, to see if he'd be free for an interview. I sent another to Sir B. He wrote me this message:

Are you ready to come here to do some things and I am not talking about having any physical contact with me but to do as I say . . . are you ready for that? You just need to trust, no questions asked and just do as told knowing I know whats best.

B

As the image of the dungeon, the wall of toys, and the colonic were rekindled, I told him I didn't think I was ready, hoping he'd invite me to another interesting party, but I never heard from him again. The dom had given up on me.

But Eric wrote back. He told me to come over: Betty was out of town. We'd have the apartment to ourselves, with no distractions.

THE PUSSY WHISPERER

Eric was in black jeans and a pec-hugging shirt that said UNDER ARMOUR. It was even tighter than the one he'd worn the first time I'd seen him. The scene seemed set for a romantic rendezvous. The lights were low; candles flickered in the corners. Trance music played at the same tranquil level as the scent of incense. My voice came out robotic: "So, you ready for the interview?"

I looked up at him—he's six feet tall—and as he told me about his day, I noticed a brass statue of a flying cock on the bookcase behind him. It almost looked like it was perched on top of his brown-curl-clad head and about to come at me. Eric was a little bit goofy, but his Virginia twang gave him an alluring sweetness. He told me kids used to make fun of his well-endowed nose; in defense, he'd tell the bullies it allowed him to please two girls at once. That tended to shut them up.

I couldn't locate an ounce of fat on his entire body. He said he'd been getting in better shape recently. The Mother of Masturbation had made him highly aware of feminine issues, he said, and it was only fair that he be in shape for women since women are expected to be in shape for men. He could sense my tension, so he got us moving around. He taught me some martial-arts-type somersaults he'd been learning at the gym to help me loosen up. We flipped forward, sideways, and backward across the blue carpet.

He said female ninjas could be especially skillful when they realized the power behind their gender. They could feign being intimidated, playing up the stereotype of the perpetually frightened female, drawing the male attacker closer so they could obliterate him.

I've always thought using my gender—puckering my lips, sticking out my chest, whispering softly—to get anything—a job, a better grade, a cut in line, a free ticket—was only making gender inequality worse. And where did a vagina get you anyway? Having a vagina got me locked in a room, stuck in a car with a sick pedophilic ice-cream man. Having a vagina made me leave addresses of interviewees with my roommates in case I wound up locked in a dungeon. It made them worry if I wasn't home on time. Because of the folds of skin between my thighs, my parents wouldn't let me walk to the corner store alone. My brothers got to. A vagina was limiting—you got stuck, locked up, left behind, made into a target. The less I acknowledged mine, the more, I imagined, I'd get to do. But those ninja girls had a different idea.

Eric plopped Indian-style on the ground and answered my questions for close to two hours.

He rolled around as he commented—did headstands, came up on his elbows, flipped from stomach to back like a pancake—reacting to each word viscerally.

Eric was basically a fitness trainer for sex, a professional lover. He had taught couples how to have better sex, deflowered unhappy virgins, brought the preorgasmic over the edge, and helped the masturbatorily timid to confidently wield a vibrator.

THE PUSSY WHISPERER

Eric's goal, through his teaching, was to help people understand their sexuality and help men become sensitive lovers. He quoted Betty to make his point: "Many men use vaginas to jack off in."

He and Betty had met eight years before. He was twenty-three and living in Virginia; she was seventy. He had read her book, *Sex for One*, and became inspired. He wanted to learn more, hands-on, from a woman who wasn't shy to try new things. He thought if a woman stimulated her clit herself, then he could be a more conscientious lover, and use more of his focus on other parts of her body. They e-mailed back and forth until Betty finally agreed to let him visit. He came up for a four-day stay and fulfilled his fantasy of having sex with a woman while she simultaneously used a Magic Wand. He soon finished school and moved in with Betty; it was supposed to be short-term, but it worked out so well that he stayed and even helped her with the research to write *Sex for Two*. Now they were nonmonogamous lovers. Their only rule was to not have sex with another person in the one-bedroom apartment while the other one was there.

Once our conversation was over, he wanted to be sure that I gave him credit in the book for his favorite line: *Sex is the engine of joy.*

"It's all yours," I promised.

So I went to the bathroom to get prepared for my trek home, but when I returned, two square silk pillows were on the floor. I kneeled down next to Eric. He said he liked the journey I was on and if there was anything he could do to help me break through my barriers, he would do it, and for free (as long as I put his name in the book). My hands got clammy; my ears caught fire. I knew Betty, my fairy godmother of physical pleasure, was behind his offer; knowing a well-intentioned woman was orchestrating it made me feel better. After all, Betty believed no woman was whole until she was aware of what turns her on.

So here we go: Eric Wilkinson, Eric Wilkinson, Eric Wilkinson.

Eric leapt up and went to the kitchen. He started blending a raspberry protein shake. Everything he did and ate had to be healthy because when his body was healthy, his orgasms would be stronger, he said. He said he'd tell me about the orgasmic diet later, but winked and told me to make sure to take my omega-3s.

"It'll give you *grrr* . . ." he said.

He paused while mixing bananas and powders and got down on the floor to demonstrate how Betty trained him to be sensitive to women. He spread his legs out like a woman in missionary and said Betty slammed her body against his for fifteen minutes so he would know the thigh fatigue a woman feels.

We slurped our shakes as we sat Indian-style across from each other. My heart pounded, and Clitty Rose was definitely on high alert. I did my cheek-biting thing and picked at a tiny bump near my hairline. It was a nervous tic, this picking thing. The bump anchored my jittery hands, kept them busily focused on my body's own geography.

"I want you to leave here tonight feeling better about yourself than when you arrived," he said. "If that happens, then we've succeeded."

As our roles changed—me from interviewer to student, him from interviewee to teacher—confidence and grace overtook him while anxiety clawed at my throat. He took my hand away from my head and told me to breathe deeply.

"See the anxiety leave your lips," he said. I breathed.

"Thank you for your trust," he said, "even if it is a tiny amount. And thank you for trusting men."

THE PUSSY WHISPERER

148

That struck something. It resonated. How did he know it would? I thought back to a man I had recently seen on the train. He was reading a book, and his thumb covered the last word in the title: *How to Live Without Fear and Wo—*. I assumed it said *Women* and was ready to write him off as a bastard, but when he saw me staring at him, his fingers fidgeted nervously, uncovering the remaining letters: *rry*. It said *Worry*. Oops.

Eric told me to touch his wrist when I was ready to move on. I assessed his symmetry as we sat. He was very well-aligned, unsurprisingly. After ten minutes of breathing, I tapped him. We moved to the bedroom. The Pilates ball was still in the corner, but this time I also noticed wooden carved dildos hanging up on the wall— now that was a conversation piece. Talking helped me take my mind off what would come next.

"Wow," I said. "Those are nice."

"Betty likes the one with the long handle," he said. "The handle makes for good control."

The television was set to Soundscapes, a station with tranquil music. He reduced the glare by placing pillows against the screen and lighting candles around Betty's dildos. The windows framed views into other high-rise bedrooms. Eric said he'd never seen anything interesting in his neighbor's windows for all the eight years he'd been there. It made him sad—and not just because he occasionally enjoyed being voyeuristic—that more people weren't getting it on across the way. He felt people routinely, to the point of habitualization, released their sexual energies into unhealthy outlets like excessive eating and attempted fulfillment by practicing materialism, as if a new sweater would somehow quench a lack of physical satisfaction, as if a hard-on could be replaced by a new car.

He politely turned away as I peeled off my shirt. I lay face-down, with my pants and bra still on. He splashed almond oil onto his hands, warmed it between his palms, and began massaging me.

"Can I touch your lower back?" he asked.

He wouldn't touch anywhere until I said he could. He gave me options every step of the way and would only go on once he got an answer from me. He said it was important for women, especially in the beginning, to know they were in control. Giving permission empowered me. I knew I had to go no further than I wanted and that I didn't have to feel guilty about blue balls at the end of the night—the focus of the evening was not to get him off. He'd already made that clear, so the pressure was off.

"Can I touch your neck?" he said.

"Yes, you may."

He blew warm air on my neck and kneaded my shoulders.

"The red pillow, the brown hair, the chopsticks in your hair," he said. "I wish I could take a photo and show you. Women would be amazed to see how beautiful they are."

He told me to listen to my sexual energy. He said to let *her* guide me through the evening. "We want *her* to feel the *grrr* . . ." he said.

Baby step by baby step. Soon I had on only my underwear and a towel across my chest. He closed his eyes as he laid it over my breasts.

"It's important to tell a woman why she's beautiful," he said. "Not just *that* she's beautiful, but specifically *why* she's beautiful."

He traced my figure along the covers and said he liked the hourglass curve of my hips, the down on the small of my back. He said my calves, which I normally describe as tumorous, were as erotic as a second pair of breasts. He told me how every woman has beauty and can be erotic in her own way. He was with a severely obese woman once and said that while she sat on top of him, she was like a cloud he could get lost in; he was immersed in her warmth.

I told Eric that one of my biggest barriers has always been when a man's face gets near *her*. I'd never wanted a guy to judge *me* by *her* stink. Clitty Rose was a trigger-happy and sensitive sensor, which caused my legs to slam shut after perceiving the slightest approach of a masculine face. Eric looked almost as if he was heartbroken due to my lack of face-to-pussy loving, so sad it appeared that I'd just told him I'd had a groom ditch me at the altar. He immediately took action.

He sat between my legs. "Once you break through," he said, "you're going to feel like you're throwing off an old stuffy coat."

He asked permission to touch my inner thighs.

"Yes."

I was losing focus; I was thinking of how I might stink, how my leg stubble might feel. He caught on right away. He took me back to my body.

"Get out of your head," he reminded me. "Breathe and feel."

He kissed my thigh and then hovered above the front triangle of my underwear.

"May I take your scent?" he asked.

Scent, come on: it was a stench, an odor. I kept breathing. We breathed together. I finally nodded and he lightly sniffed. He brought his head back up and told me what he had found. He said I was mild and mostly smelled of fabric softener. I breathed a sigh of relief. He asked if he could take my scent again. I let him. He used his chin, forehead, and that long proboscis of his to stimulate me. I found it easier to keep my focus because I wasn't thinking of all the things that would pop up if we were trying to develop a relationship. I wasn't wondering if he had the right job, if he'd be a good father, if he was into me or just my pussy, or if he'd call me later if my pussy wasn't up to par.

Eric looked up. I propped up my head and gazed past my belly to him, framed between the V made by my two bent legs. He smiled. He brought his face near to mine—his nose just below my nostrils—and then he introduced me to me.

"This is you," he said. "Your scent is bright. If smells could have a light, yours would twinkle."

I coughed out a laugh. Something significant had just happened; maybe an old coat hadn't busted off me, but an old sweatshirt—a layer, at least—certainly had. This signaled the beginning of a truce between Clitty Rose and me. She had an aroma, but I wouldn't call it a stink exactly.

ERIC WILKINSON, ERIC WILKINSON, ERIC WILKINSON.

"If we stop right now," I said. "I'm going to be very proud of myself."

He didn't make me second-guess myself by asking if I was sure. He only asked if I wanted to cuddle before I left. I did. We talked, reflected, and wound down from the evening. He said he looked forward to breaking through more barriers with me, if I wanted.

He pecked me on the lips. I smiled and laughed in the deliciousness of being treated like a princess. Was I a slut, or an adventurer going deeper into myself than I'd ever gone before? There was a split-second when I thought of my brother: Is this the part where people would think I was a whore? Oh, well, it didn't matter. As I walked down the hall toward the elevator, I thanked Betty for her generous loan. My gender was part of my identity, just like my shape, size, and mind. Knowing my femininity wouldn't be abusing it, and suppressing it wouldn't make it go away, but embracing it might allow me to go ninja-style.

THE PUSSY WHISPERER

When I gave my roommates the details the following morning, they looked at me first with worry—"He what?"—and then wonderment.

"I think there's a market for a pull-string Eric doll," Leigh said, mimicking pulling a cord. "'You are beautiful. Your scent twinkles. You are beautiful. Your scent twinkles.'"

Ursula laughed. "I want a boyfriend like that."

"He's available," I said.

"I said *like* that," she said. "I don't want to date a guy who's also dating the seventy-eight-year-old Mother of Masturbation."

"Point taken," I said.

Leigh was still churning the idea of a sex surrogate in her mind, and it wasn't necessarily an easy concept. "I get it," Leigh said, "but I just don't get it. How could you be with someone who you don't like, like romantically?"

What about one-night stands, I said. "How can people go home with a stranger and actually screw?" I asked. "That's no stranger than going to someone's home to learn sex techniques. And at least Eric has my well-being in mind instead of just getting himself off."

I was so persuasive that I almost convinced myself that the situation was normal.

"I still don't get it," said Leigh.

Okay, maybe I didn't either. But I liked it.

I called up Zola the next day. I wanted to tell her everything and have her help me make sense of what had happened. As we slid into the booth at the Galaxy Diner, she gave me a Tantra lesson of the day. Each time I sat down, she told me, I should rock back and forth a little until I registered exactly where Clitty Rose settled on my seat.

"You'll have awareness of your body that way," she said, rocking back and forth and making little groans. "And it feels great."

I told her about what had happened with Eric.

"He introduced me to me," I told Zola. She bounced up and down in the pleather booth; it squeaked as she clapped her hands above her head.

"He's your own sacred whore!" she said. "That's so hot!"

"What?" I said. "Explain this to me, please."

She told me that for many thousands of years, before prudery became mainstream, "prostitute" and "whore" were respectful titles, like "reverend" is today. She said the whores lived in sacred temples and were highly trained in the art of sex. Basically, they were sex professors. As simple and innocuous as employing someone to wash your car today, in the age Zola called the Goddess Era, people offered up cash in order to polish up their sexual proficiency. She said the students would learn how to reach higher orgasmic potentials, harness sexual energies, open up, let go, and even heal emotionally. Eric, in the temple of Betty, was bringing back an ancient ritual, she said.

"Does that make me a whore too?" I asked.

"Whore's not a bad thing," she reiterated.

She told me there were a lot of things that people say are bad that are actually good. She gave childbirth as an example. The pain, she says, is a societal interpretation; it can be traced all the way back to the Garden of Eden. "God said to Eve that she was getting kicked out of a dope-ass place and, P.S., you're going to cry and writhe in pain when you give birth to human beings," she explained. Zola said the uterine contractions that occur during childbirth are very similar to the ones during orgasm. "The pain of childbirth," Zola said, "is actually a good-ass, Masters and Johnson, uterine-contraction orgasm!"

THE VERB'S NOT A WORD

I needed to get an external hard drive for my computer. Noam had always been good at these types of errands. Remember Noam? I hope you remember him from his brief cameo in Peru; we'd met in the coffee shop where I worked. He was tall and built like a line-backer, with chocolate-syrup-colored skin that he'd inherited from his Bolivian roots. His deep voice rumbled as if there were an ice machine in his throat. We'd been in contact for the past few years and had had a few minor romantic run-ins since his move to New York. We never did more than kiss because it seemed that despite our mutual attraction, our rendezvous always went defective. If you recall, our one attempted kiss in Peru was botched when a gigantic crucified Jesus paraded past during some religious procession. The last time I had seen him, the pattern had persisted.

A writer friend had told me that a book delving into female sexuality wouldn't be properly researched without watching a Catherine Breillat film. They're all about female sexuality, he said. I had invited Noam over, thinking we could catch up over a dimly lit room and a rental. I should have known better. Breil-lat's a French director—you know, the bleak and morbid kind. *Fat Girl* was about two sisters. One was fat and ate all the time; the other was skinny and got it on with rich college boys. Noam and I were jiving on each other a bit—Clitty Rose even sent up a faint tingle—but we didn't touch; we were both the fat girl, eating away our sexual tension with handfuls of falafel. Then the skinny girl got murdered and the fat girl got raped; she looked disconcertingly satisfied at having her cherry popped as blood pooled around her sister's neck. It wasn't a feel-good flick. It left me with the heebie-jeebies and, I'm pretty sure, Noam with a soft dick.

A couple weeks later, after scanning so many hard drives that I was seeing them on the inside of my eyelids, Noam and I went out to dinner at a French bistro. He had the hanger steak, and I had skate over navy beans.

"Isn't it weird," I said. "If you think about it, almost every guy's face you see has had pussy in it."

Noam looked around the restaurant. "That's not weird," he said. "It's weirder that people wear hats and sweatshirts."

"What do you mean?"

"It's a much more natural thing to have pussy in your mouth than a hat on your head," he said. "Everyone's first moment of life, they have a mouthful of pussy."

"Not Cesarean-section babies," I countered.

"Were you a C-section baby?"

"Yes."

"Figures."

We ended up in his apartment. We hooked up my new external hard drive on my laptop to see if it worked. He poured me a glass of wine as the drive revved up.

We got kind of close and were both a little tipsy. He asked me if he could try my twinkle for dessert.

Hmmm.

I'd just read in the book *Woman: An Intimate Geography* by Natalie Angier that the pH of a healthy pussy is 3.8 to 4.5, matching the acidity of red wine—and I knew Noam was a connoisseur of the beverage.

Besides, someone's nose had just been down there, and he hadn't spontaneously combusted, right? I could do this. Here was my chance to show myself I'd made headway (so to speak). I'd drunk enough that I was like an agoraphobic on Xanax going to the market for the first time—obviously having reservations, but sedated enough to give it a try.

I leaned against a side of his sofa. He almost burned his foot on a candle as he contorted to fit me. As if my membrane could soak up the traces of fermented grape on his palette, I felt my outlook become even blurrier. In that position, I always expected the man to seem as distant as the antlike people on the sidewalk seen from a skyscraper, but he wasn't. I could clearly see the cowlick swirl in his hair—even touch it. It was a nice sensation, but it lasted about one minute before my thinking went retrograde. I suddenly desired to diagram our activities in an overly obtuse and unhelpful way, like my linguistic teachers insisted I do to compound-laden sentences in college.

See, I like the penis. I have a healthy respect for the organ. I might even have the desire for one (or who knows, maybe a couple?) to play a more stable role in my life at some point, but that hose-shaped apparatus is misclassified; it's not just a noun. The intention behind its structure is not stationary—the penis is implicitly action-oriented—and very quickly takes on verblike qualities: to poke, to prod, to prick, to penis.

I seem to excel at making a jovial mood decline toward dismal disaster. With Eric, it was decided that I'd have all the attention, but here I felt the bulge that was Noam's verb against my leg and instantly started guilting myself for letting it linger in its rigidity—a verb must happen, the diagram must branch off and grow in a direction. Now, I'd like to touch the penis, play with it, but there's a snowball effect that occurs. Touching the penis is like starting a sentence: there's a mandatory moment of tangible punctuation (I learned fragments are cause for bad grades). I wanted options, but the mythological idea of blue balls began to hang over my head like a piñata. The party wouldn't be a success unless it was busted.

And what if it led to sex? I wasn't ready for six and a half on my list; only four more and I'd have to take my socks off to have enough digits to count them all up. When I thought of the number of men that I'd been with, I saw a pie chart dividing me into slices. The more men I was with, the smaller the slice of me I could give. At what point would there be nothing left?

I could no longer hold off my habitual reaction. My legs snapped shut on Noam—scissor-style. He fell to the side of the couch, accidentally knocking over the hard drive; the plug ripped out of my computer. Both appliances went dead. I packed up my damaged devices and went back to Brooklyn, head a little lower than when I'd departed five hours earlier.

Man, did I feel shitty. I did not feel good at all. The worst part was that I felt worse for Noam's unsatiated weenie than I felt for my partially consumed pussy. Sorry, Clitty Rose.

I called up Fiona at one in the morning and began to tell her what happened.

"He ate you out?!" she interrupted. She sounded proud, like she did when I got my first bra.

THE VERB'S NOT A WORD

158

"Ahh," I said, "don't call it that, and no, not really. Well, kind of. He tried to, but . . ."

I told her it didn't go as desired and started talking to her about the number of men that she'd been with. I told her about the slices theory.

"Oh no," she said, disagreeing. "Each man doesn't take anything away. Each sexual experience only adds."

That was a positive outlook. We tried to remember, together, how many sex partners she'd had. It took about twenty minutes to get them all down on paper.

"Twenty-three," she said. "Yep, twenty-three. No, wait, do girls count?"

"Sure."

"Then twenty-six," she said. "Perfect! One for each year."

And as it turns out, she had just added the twenty-sixth that week. In what seemed like a nanosecond after breaking the divorce news to Pedro, she'd already met someone new. He was on tour with her. Benjamin was a musician; he'd sit in the orchestra pit each evening, staring up at her as she danced. She'd stopped reading *Eat, Pray, Love*—she said it got boring—and moved on to Ayn Rand's *The Fountainhead*, per Benjamin's suggestion.

"Mara," she said, "I've never felt this way before. He just *gets* me."

She was at it again, her pattern. I was mid–eye roll when I suddenly aborted the retinal arc and started questioning my exasperation. I began wondering how she managed to find so many guys who were right for her—not just right, but *perfect* for her—while absolutely zero seemed even an iota plausible for me. Maybe she's not a commitment-addict after all, but there's just a fate we're each born with: Numerous people have "the one"; others, like Fiona, have "the many"; and a few of us have "the none."

HERE A TWAT. THERE A TWAT.
EVERYWHERE A TWAT-TWAT.

I was feeling kind of low after the Noam encounter. I wanted to get my ass in gear, motivate myself a little, so I contacted fifty-four-year-old Dr. R. J. Noonan, founder of the now-in-remission Consortium for Sex Research in Space, to speak to him about orgasms in space. I'm not sure why I thought this was a good idea; I was getting rather ahead of myself. But if humans ruined the Earth and were living in space stations by the time I got this freaking orgasm, I wanted to know if it'd be as hot of an experience without gravity. "They'd be less intense because of lower blood pressure," he said, "but more necessary because of all the stress." That's a bummer, I guess—but I suppose it's also one more good reason not to destroy the Earth.

Serendipitously, I found out R. J. Noonan would also be at a sexuality conference I'd signed up to attend—and he'd be a speaker, no less.

See, I was about to leave the city. I was sick of making a mess in my own backyard. I'd been in touch with a lot of sex professionals throughout the country, so I used those contacts to design a sexual odyssey to fit conveniently and affordably around my customary trip home for Thanksgiving. I was going to Indianapolis for the sex conference, then home to San Diego for Thanksgiving, then to San Francisco (which Annie Sprinkle calls the clit of the country) for a week of orgasm immersion, and finally on to the northernmost tip of the California woods for Orgasm Camp with the family Racheli Cherwitz of OneTaste had told me about. Because they wanted to remain unidentified in order to maintain their privacy, I began referring to them as the Orgasm People. I spoke briefly with a woman named Samantha about their secluded orgasmic lifestyle; she told me their "family" focuses their lifework on researching orgasm—they have more than one hundred years of combined orgasm research experience. I signed up for a three-day sensuality course. I didn't know anything about what I'd learn, except that there would be one section called OIC: Observation of Intense Coming. It lasted for a full hour. And it was not like tag-team style; one woman actually did all the coming, all by herself—sixty minutes of continuously coming. Fucking crazy, right?

So, back to serendipity. It was serendipitous that Dr. R. J. Noonan, who goes by Ray, was attending the sex convention because it turned out that his lecture partner had to stay home and he had an extra bed at the Hyatt. I didn't have a place to stay yet; I'd pondered couch-surfing, but all my friends told me that was sketch. Ray told me he was hoping to get some action—it was the first time he'd had his own room at a sex conference in what seemed like decades—but that he would ponder letting me stay anyway.

"We could have a top-secret phrase," I said, "and if you get lucky, you can text me and I'll know to stay in the lobby for a while."

He said he'd get back to me later.

When I met up with Zola to say good-bye, she prepared me for whomever I might run into on my trip. First she ranked the nationalities based on their head-giving receptivity: "Guys from Chile don't. Argentina does. Dominican Republic does it. Trinidad does not. Israel, from quite a few reports, does not, but sure enjoys the BJs," she said. She brushed her hair behind her ears and took a bite of a seared Japanese dumpling drowned in ponzu vinaigrette. As she chewed she moaned as if a Dominican were under the table and then continued with her thought: "If they're not going to eat it, then I'm sorry, beat it!"

Then she warned me to make men brush their teeth before going down on Clitty Rose, especially after beer: the foreign yeast can throw your own fungus out of balance and land you a date with Monistat, she said.

Unfortunately, after that interesting, yet slightly off-putting conversational nugget, I had to break some bad news to Zola: I had to tell her what I thought of the DVD, *Divine Nectar*, she'd given me on our first visit. What I had to say only demonstrated that I was not a highly evolved woman in touch with her inner sacred goddess and yoni portal. I watched the video on my sofa with the cup of coffee I always get from the corner deli. I pressed play and immediately got queasy when a man started filling a chalice with his wife's ejaculate. Because that's what this film was about: women reclaiming their ability to ejaculate. Did you know women can ejaculate? I actually spit out my coffee, and I ALWAYS finish my coffee.

I'm telling you, this movie would be a great instrument for a bulimic. Even now, just thinking about it, I feel like I'm going to puke up breakfast. Zola didn't seem offended. She told me about her female ejaculation experiences and said an ejaculatory orgasm can be better than therapy. "It's so deep and so real, a release like none other," she said. I believed her. I handed back the DVD, contritely.

HERE A TWAT. THERE A TWAT. EVERYWHERE A TWAT-TWAT.

Zola gave me the number of her friend Satya, who lived in San Francisco. Satya called herself an undercover goddess and also worked as a *dakini*. Zola told me that if I was ready to learn more while out West, I should make an appointment. Zola hugged me, squeezed me—all her sex energy poking at me—and said she'd be waiting patiently for all the stories when I got back to the City.

The day before I left, I had one last therapy appointment. I looked at Rori. Rori looked at me. She pulled the bangs out of her eyes. I rubbed my hands together. She crossed her legs. I patted my bangs to be sure they were all pointing down, in formation.

After our fidget-fest finished, I started telling her about my latest dream. A steel beaded chain hung between people's legs. When tugged, it clicked on the orgasmic switch, just like it would the light under a lampshade. Everyone spasmed until it was pulled again. But someone had cut off my chain.

"How are other things going?" she asked.

"What do you mean by *other* things?" I asked. "What other things?"

"Exactly," she said.

She warned me that my head was too much in my vagina. She said I needed to take some time for my whole self—shopping, seeing friends, a museum.

"I don't want to objectify you," she said, "but it's hard, because you're objectifying yourself. You're not just a vulva."

But whatever my work was, I made into my life. Vulva was my work, so inevitably vulva had become my life. Maybe she was right—I'd turned into a twat. I got my version of the ejaculatory release; I started crying, just bawling, tears careening down my face.

I called my mom as I walked out of the office.

"Mom," I said, clearly distraught, "my therapist told me I'm too single-minded. She says that I've turned into one big giant twat, a twat that sits on her couch."

"You know," my mom said, "finding a partner can really help you calm down. A man can add balance, like Ken—"

I hung up on her.

Atman, my crotch guru, couldn't even help; he told me I'd figure it all out if I boozed it up. "We need something to walk and breathe naturally," he said. "One shot of scotch, whiskey, or something."

Tell me something I didn't know.

Then he gave me a free scone, grabbed my face, and gave me a big fat kiss on my lips. I felt dazed by the onslaught of Atman.

"You will bring back something very healthy from your trip," he said.

What was he, a freaking prophetic wizard now—a guru wasn't enough? Why didn't he just whip out a crystal ball?

Atman's little pep talk didn't work, so I went back to moping and taking food "samples" from the Whole Foods salad bar. The habit was so obnoxious that I couldn't even talk to Rori about it. I was like Winona Ryder, all klepto, and one day they'd catch me scarfing down Shanghai dumplings in the paper towel section, pretending I was digging to the back for the freshest roll. They'd look at my wallet and see that it was full of cash, and then interrogate me and discover it came from prostituting my feet for an hour. Then they'd call me a whore. *The whore is sacred, didn't you hear?*

When I got home, the bad didn't stop. As I packed that evening, one of the cats vomited inside my green and gold flats, adding a hint of tuna-tinged fishiness to their rubbery smell. Ursula attacked the pair with spritzes of Febreze, but still . . . Then I checked my e-mail and my Nerve profile. I'd been on two more dates for the hell of it, nothing special. One tried to lift me up after our drink

HERE A TWAT. THERE A TWAT. EVERYWHERE A TWAT-TWAT.

and I had to duck and then sprawl on the pavement to avoid his grasp. I suspected that my other date had been gay. I'm not saying he was—I fully admit to having had faulty gay-dar in the past—but my gay-dar kept bleeping louder than I could ignore as he had described, in detail, the way he'd picked out his new teak desk. Then, as I opened my dating profile, I could see Joe had been viewing me; that was a first in a month (not that I was checking). I checked out his picture. We were both online. We were having a virtual stare-down, probably one he wasn't privy to. I wanted him to want me. I wanted him to call me and say he was sorry. After that, I could say, "See, I told you. I told you you'd feel this way."

I walked toward my balcony to see The Collector's hoard, thinking it must be up to at least the second story by now. I leaned over; I bent my head down. The backyard was pristine. The semi must have come and swept it all away again. Even my literary conceit crumbled away in the wake of a bad day. Literary devices were as fickle as my clit.

At least Ray Noonan called; he said he'd be happy to donate his empty bed at the sexuality conference to my cause. I was more than ready to get out of town and have some sex researchers tell me what was wrong with me.

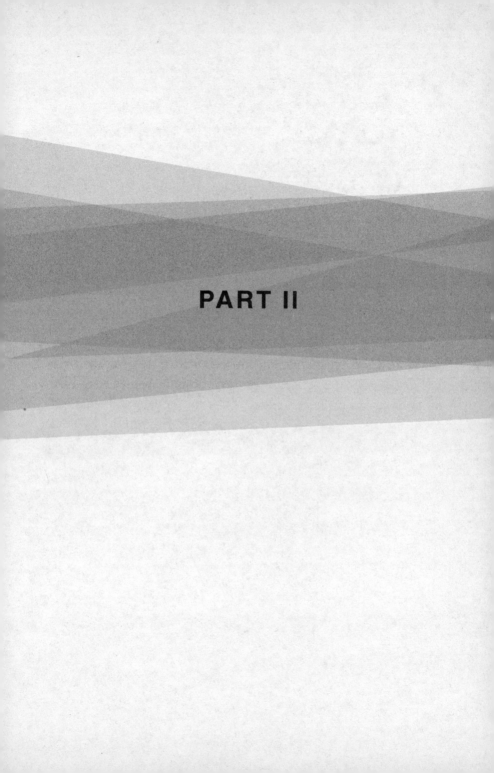

PART II

EVOLUTION USED TO BE A GENIUS

Ray and I attended the welcoming reception for the fiftieth anniversary convention of the SSSS, the Society for the Scientific Study of Sexuality. "She's famous for sexual assault and rape," Ray said, pointing out a star of sex research as she passed us in the Hyatt ballroom. "He's a specialist in sexual compulsivity," he said. "She named the G-spot," pointing to someone else. I wasn't the average attendee; there were scientists, educators, therapists, and even some sex workers. They were there to present papers and give talks about recent studies. I was an outsider, but it was perfect; I had a whole conference full of captive sex experts.

I mingled. I met the guy who writes the pamphlets for Planned Parenthood—I figured that must be like *New Yorker* writer status in the sex education world. I pumped his hand and tried to suck up with a compliment: great ponytail.

Most of the people at the conference were older. The majority were somewhere in their forties to sixties—the decades straddling either side of my parents' age. There were a couple pockets filled

168

with my generation, but it seemed that the generation that had ripened in tandem with the sexual revolution had laid their claim on sex—academic sex, criminal sex, fetish sex, romantic sex, righteous sex, same sex, sex expressed by graphs and decimal points, sex sex sex. It was their domain.

When not inside, Ray puffed his pipe, which made him smell sweet, spicy, and yellow—yes, yellow. Since we were sharing a room, I wondered if all my clothes would smell yellow by the time I packed up for California. At the conference, Ray was presenting his 1,419-page book called *The Continuum Complete International Encyclopedia of Sexuality*. He was a sex nerd. He knew all sorts of weird sex factoids, and he spouted them at random moments: fifty to eighty percent of spouses cheat; deeply religious women are the most sexually satisfied; dentists are the professionals, he'd heard, who were most likely to have affairs with their patients. He said he knew his daughter was gay before she did. I wondered if I was gay and he knew but wasn't telling me. I wanted to ask him, but I didn't know what I would do with the information—dealing with one pussy was enough for me at the moment.

In the morning, Ray coiffed his hair into a shiny cresting mass above his forehead. He wore a beat-up leather bomber jacket; I figured it'd been around since the late sixties, just like the bouffant mustache hiding half his smile. He missed the sixties and seventies. It was free love then. Now we were in an unsexy time, a time when people thought physical education teachers were properly equipped to teach sex education to the masses, as if being nimble enough to roll a condom on a cucumber was the most challenging part of the sexual equation—not pleasure, not ethics, not romance, and certainly not variation, only rubber. Sex was about rubber, the unfurling of rubber.

Thanks for Coming

The first day didn't yield as much as I'd hoped for. I went on a bus tour to the Kinsey Institute in Bloomington, Indiana. I thought of it as a pilgrimage. I couldn't understand my orgasm without bowing down to the altar of Dr. Alfred Kinsey. During the fifties, he had brought sexuality into the national conversation by interviewing eighteen thousand people about their sex practices and publishing the results in thick books popularly called the Kinsey Reports. They revealed that much more went on in Americans' bedrooms than actual penis-to-cooch intercourse, which was revelatory at the time. He put a little gay into everyone by showing that people's sexualities weren't black or white. Kinsey concluded that the only unnatural sex act was that which you could not perform.

We had only an hour when we arrived, hardly enough time to take a decent gander. Most of the sex people took a brief peek but spent the majority of the time taking photos or buying sweatshirts, mugs, and postcards with the Kinsey Institute insignia. I hoped they weren't practicing the retail therapy that Eric, my sacred whore, had talked about, making up for lack of sexual interaction with purchasing potency. What good would the sex people be if they couldn't satisfy their own carnal cravings?

Then I ran into Julia Heiman, the present director of the Kinsey Institute. In the seventies, with two colleagues, she had written the book *Becoming Orgasmic*. I told her that I had it at home—but not that I hadn't made it past chapter two. I already knew I needed help; her self-help book only belabored the point and depressed me.

I asked her about overcoming my sexual inhibitions. "Inhibitions actually can be very protective," she said. "In sex, women have more to lose. Women, remember, in spite of contraception—which is a pretty recent development in human history—women can get pregnant. The fact that women at this point in our evolutionary history may be more programmed to be inhibited is to their advantage." It helps us be more careful in choosing our partners, she said.

Evolution seemed so smart, especially when Darwin got all ranty about his finches, but one thing it didn't think through was adding a fifth gear. Evolution was too damn slow. We should have an extra finger poking out of our navels by now, a digit specifically designed to unbutton the flies on our jeans. Inhibitions should have shed themselves after Margaret Sanger's birth control activism in the early 1900s. Fucking evolution—it used to be a genius.

I had more orgasm questions, but I got derailed when I couldn't hide my true curiosity: How had her last name, Heiman, affected her career? It wasn't the right spelling, but it sounded the same as the piece of tissue that rests in the vaginal canal as an obstruction to virginal penetration. You couldn't ignore the irony. And that's where my interview with that particular celebrity of sex research ended.

(I even followed up later with e-mail. She has yet to get back to me, for the record.)

As I exited, the buses already throttling outside for our return, a framed sketch on the wall caught my attention. It was one from Japan called *Cunt Hell of Great Searing Heat*. It looked like a *Braveheart* battle scene, but all the charging warriors had vagina heads with angry-looking labial sneers. I bet Clitty Rose could get pissed like that. In fact, I thought, she will be if I don't figure this shit out.

When I got back to the hotel, Ray and I went out for dinner. I sipped a beer and leaned my forehead on my hand. He wanted to help me. "Babies masturbate in utero," he said. It had been documented in sonograms. Boy fetuses grab their baby cocks, so he assumed fetal girls touched themselves, too. "You probably had an orgasm in the womb." He smiled, trying to cheer me up. I nodded, as I looked at the menu. He told me that women have nocturnal orgasms just like men have nocturnal emissions—wet dreams. "You've probably had one while you were sleeping," he said, mollifying me. I was impressed, but still: "That's not the kind I want," I told him.

I thought of Alzheimer's disease. My maternal grandmother had that before I got the chance to know the *her* she was before she forgot who she was. She'd sit in a rocking chair, rocking back and forth while watching *I Love Lucy* reruns and thumbing smooth beads. She died not remembering one come she had ever had, I bet.

"What good's a come if you don't remember it?" I said.

TURNING YELLOW

There's nothing like talk of genital ulcers in the morning to make cheese Danishes lose their appeal. It's hard to make sex a boring subject, but it was like these researchers actually went out of their way to make it dry. I complained to a nearby sexologist. "If you think this is dry," he said, a little defensive, "you should see the AIDS conferences."

Ray already knew the secret of conferences; he went to them so he could use the hotel swimming pool. There were PowerPoint presentations, handouts, and long droning lectures. I kept slipping out ten minutes into each discussion. I had things to do, but once I got into the hall, I wondered what they were. It occurred to me that maybe it wasn't only inhibitions but also impatience that led to my anorgasmia—an unwillingness to see an activity all the way to the end. I'm easily distracted.

Like when I saw a giant kilt-clad man walk by. I stopped him and asked him about his thoughts on the female orgasm. "Not much," he said. "The man's is what I'm interested in." He guffawed a movie villain's guffaw, a guffaw that sent shock waves through the floor as he lumbered away.

I finally decided I had to do something drastic. I went to a lecture about female sexuality. I munched my cheek, managing to stay all the way to the end. They passed around a microphone for questions and comments. I decided it was now or never. Twenty sex professionals were my prisoners.

I hate speaking in public.

Microphones are worse than smelling yellow. I'd rather smell all kinds of yellow—smoky yellow, puke yellow, diarrhea yellow—than hear my voice go up in decibel levels. Fiona lives and gets paid for her voice being amplified into as many decibels as possible—the more far-reaching, the better. I've never understood it.

"Hi," I said, my words sounding like they were hooked up to a life support system, thump-thump-thumping between syllables. "I'm Mara Altman, and I'm trying to have my first orgasm. If any of you have any pointers, please let me know."

No one said anything. Maybe there was a chuckle. Maybe there was even an appalled cackle. I couldn't tell; I was deafened by my extreme desire to just be a puddle of yellow. When I refocused, everyone was filing out of the room. One woman came up to me, holding out her book, *Women's Sexualities*. "There's a chapter on orgasm," she said. "It's only fifteen dollars, a good price for students."

She wasn't the first to try to sell her book to me. That's what people did when I asked for interviews—these sex people just told me to buy their books. Everyone was touting something because almost everyone there had a published how-to on better sex. It was annoying, but knowing there was a market out there did make me feel a little better. It meant I wasn't the only one who sucked at sex.

I grimaced.

She plopped her book back in her bag and walked away.

Glasses were the most distinctive thing about the gray-haired woman who approached me next. Her name was Elizabeth Rae Larson. I had seen the first ten minutes of one of her lectures; I had almost stayed longer because she used curse words.

We sat in a corner of quiet. She said she'd been a sexologist for decades. She fought for sexual rights and equality during the sixties. We plunged right into an interview.

"How can I find my orgasm?" I said.

"The women's movement," she said, "said that the orgasm is positive for women, something they ought to have. But it moved from being an opportunity to a mandate. It created social pressure that says something's wrong with you if you don't."

"Exactly. So what's wrong with me?"

"People overvalue orgasm," she reiterated. "They go looking for an orgasm instead of pleasure. Look for pleasure first; that will lead you where you want to go."

We continued talking for a while, but I had heard all I could bear. I think she was saying orgasm didn't matter anymore. Of course she was saying that; she had already gotten as many as she wanted.

Larson left me with my bubble popped. Not only did I not have my orgasm, but she was telling me I wasn't even allowed to say there was something wrong with me. As I walked back toward the main hall, I ran into the woman who'd offered to sell me her book an hour before. She held it out to me, looking somewhat concerned.

"Why don't you just take it?" she said. "I don't want to carry it home anyway."

She signed the title page and handed it to me.

"Good luck," she said and turned away.

THE GREEN THING THAT'S ACTUALLY

PURPLE, WHICH MIGHT ALSO BE THE KEY

The rumors couldn't be true. Orgasms still mattered. Dr. Komisaruk proved it. He was at the conference to receive an award, along with his coauthors, for their book *The Science of Orgasm*. Now would that be happening if orgasm were passé? I didn't think so.

I didn't know he'd be there, but we ran into each other in the hall. He caught me in the corner, flipping through my new book.

"Mara!" he said. "Mara!"

He leaned toward me, his lips in a pucker headed directly for my cheek. I'm glad he extracted himself safely; I've always had a fear someone might lodge too deeply into my epidermal quicksand, getting stuck in the desert of my jowl. He whisked me away to the lobby bar. We downed some Sauvignon Blanc. Although we hadn't talked in two months, he still clearly cared about my project. He said I was brave. He said I was the Holden Caulfield of orgasms.

"It's a coming-of-age story," he said, laughing at his own word play.

I imagined myself in a field of rye, catching orgasms—undulating like wind-mangled bubbles—in butterfly nets.

"I still want you to be a participant in the study," said Dr. Komisaruk of the fMRI orgasm work he was doing. When that orgasm materialized, he wanted me to be able to see it sparking in my brain.

"I'd love to," I said, starting to Kegel in my seat. I was feeling shameful about my progress. Nothing had happened yet.

"It's just so hard to get funding," he said. He'd spent much of the previous months filling out grant applications and had gotten nothing back in return. "There's no value placed on pleasure in this country."

I remembered that line from months ago.

He had to go. He was busy. Orgasm was work to him. Before hugging me good-bye, he asked if I'd made any headway.

"It'll come," I said, hoping he didn't register my uncertainty.

That's when I decided I had to stop procrastinating and get my vibrator. It'd been two months since Dr. Komisaruk banged our dinner table, telling me it was the key. I had the keyhole; I needed the key. I went up to the main hall again, where tables were lined up. Vendors hawked products, everything from DVDs to dildos to applications for doctoral degrees.

One woman had been desperately peddling aphrodisiac oils. Her company was called Good Love. "Indian spice," she'd call out, bombarding the passersby with a slosh of oil as they tried to jolt past. "If you change the smell, you change the love."

I'd been avoiding her too, but now I figured the vibrators on her table might be the only things here that could really help me.

As I approached her table, she turned an oil bottle upside down to coordinate with the arrival of my wrists. "I'm a lovologist," she said, shaking oil onto my skin. "I don't say I sell sex products. I say I sell LOVE products, and that's because I really believe sex is the glue we were given to hold relationships together. It's not just this free-for-all where people end up getting hurt. That's not what sex is really for."

She presented herself as a warrior of eros, waging a losing battle for love. It must have been quite a fight. She looked war-torn and bedraggled. She had bags under her eyes as well as bedhead. She spoke quickly, like an auctioneer. If she stopped, I feared she'd plunk to the ground and start waving her love oil brochure like a white flag. Surrender.

"Do you study sexology?" I asked.

"I've been married twenty-five years," she said. "I study it everyday."

She kept droning on about love—she had a good take on it, I think—but I wasn't in the mood for love.

"Everyone wants it more than anything and people don't realize it's a huge amount of work to love somebody," she said, as she tried to smudge more meanderers with her love potion. "I didn't invent it," she called out after them. "I just bottled it."

She looked back at me. She rubbed a new odor onto my wrist and sniffed it as she spoke. "The issue is always in yourself," she said. "It's not in your relationship. It's not like being with someone else is going to fix your issues, does that make sense?"

"I'm working on my issues," I said.

"Welcome to the world, honey!" she said.

"I haven't had an orgasm yet," I said. "That's one of them."

"WHAT?" she said. "You haven't? You need to buy some love oil. No, some lube. No, wait, you *have* a vibrator, right?"

"No."

My lovologist picked up a small purple device. It fit perfectly in the palm of her cupped hand. "This will give you your first orgasm!" she said.

THE GREEN THING THAT'S ACTUALLY PURPLE

I took it in my hands. She explained that it was green.

"No," I said. "It's purple."

"No, it's green," she said. She meant environmentally. Instead of using up batteries, it charged in an outlet like a cell phone. It had sixteen speeds. It also came in a cute little black silk drawstring bag—so many sex things came in silk drawstring bags. Maybe I needed to buy a silk drawstring bag big enough for my whole body.

"Be clear about what it is you want," she said. "You have this idea that there's a prince who is going to meet all your needs. Forget about it, it's not true. Realize you're going to give up some things you think you want for the things you really want."

Before I could tell her I didn't want to want, she'd already written up the receipt—the vibrator was one hundred dollars, and she threw in some free lube samples—and began splashing oils onto other attendees' hands.

It was the green part of the vibrator that really got me. I wasn't just helping myself; I was helping the world—environmentally conscious self-screwing.

It was the last night. We had a final reception and auction at the Heron Gallery. Someone bid more than one hundred dollars for earrings made of Dalkon Shields, a contraceptive intrauterine device (IUD) that was taken off the market for causing infertility and infection in women. Despicable purchase, I thought. Then the woman tried them on. For a mass killer, they really looked quite dainty and feminine dangling from her lobes. I wanted a pair.

I went back to the hotel room early. Ray had been busy talking to a woman, and I was fully prepared to be kicked out of the room later on. I wanted that for Ray, but when the door creaked open at about one-thirty in the morning, Ray was alone. He didn't get lucky.

He lay in his bed. I lay in mine. It was dark. We were both on our backs, looking up at the ceiling. I felt like I was in elementary school, having a slumber party—Mom says lights out, but you keep on talking.

We talked about the conference a bit. I told him the conference was kind of helpful—at least I had bought my first vibrator. I'd be jilling off soon, as Zola called it.

"If you want," he said, "I'll have sex with you."

I didn't know what to say. I couldn't get upset, even though it was my initial reaction. It was a sweet offer, I guess. He said it like he'd offer to rub out the knots in someone's achy back. That's how casual sex could be for him. I had to decline, though; the whole idea was just a little awkward. One sacred whore, I thought, was enough for the moment.

"That's nice," I said, "but I've got that vibrator now."

"Okay," he said, sincerely. "Just making sure."

Then we continued to talk until three-thirty in the morning. We went on to one of his favorite subjects: the sexual revolution. He told me about how he and an old girlfriend used to organize orgies. Hearing him talk about it, sex started to sound like a reminiscent thing, a nostalgic thing, something for photo albums and old journal entries. I was almost sad. Sex sounded done.

He paused for a while and then told me his theory, the one he seemed to be holding out for.

"The sixties to seventies wasn't the only sexual revolution, you know?" he said. He said there was also one during the 1920s.

"It's only natural that there will be another," he said. "They come in forty-year intervals."

His voice lightened as he added it all up. "The next one should begin in 2010," he said. "Perfect!"

In that case, I promised myself, I'd be ready.

THE GREEN THING THAT'S ACTUALLY PURPLE

PLAYING HOUSE

I had a problem. I still had two nights in Indianapolis, but the conference was over. I'd booked extra nights just in case some big-name sexologist decided they just *had* to have dinner with me to divulge all their deepest orgasmic insights.

That didn't happen.

Ray left. I was roomless.

I went online to couchsurfing.com. The site lists people who offer their sofa, for free, in all different states and countries. I contacted women; none answered me. I contacted a twenty-nine-year-old named Cliff. He had a sofa available. We talked on the phone. He sounded all right. His voice was a little nasally. I usually trust nasal. So far, no one with a squeak to their voice has ever done me wrong.

Cliff picked me up at the Hyatt in his blue pickup truck. He said he would have brought the M3 BMW, but it looked like it was about to rain and he'd just waxed it. "It's my baby," he said. "Got to keep it safe in the garage."

I checked him out. He wasn't my type—he called his car his baby. I had wanted him to be my type. That would have been fun if he were my type. But what was my type?

He said he hated Indiana. He had just moved there. He was an accountant. He hated his job. He didn't have friends yet. He had a bald spot.

I wanted to touch his bald spot.

We arrived at his house. We rented the movie *Mr. Brooks*. We watched it that evening. It was about a rich and successful man who has a secret life as a serial killer. Not the best movie to watch with a stranger.

We went to bed, each a little wary of the other.

He was already at work when I woke up. The yellow stank on me; it had stuck on me. Yellow was all over. I washed it down the shower drain. I was happy to finally have some space to myself. It was a cute house. I sat on the sofa. I went for a walk. I sat on the sofa some more.

I got a little lonesome. I waited. I waited on the sofa for Cliff to get home. I paced back and forth; it was already seven-thirty p.m. Where was Cliff?

About an hour later, he opened the door. I was happy he had finally arrived. I felt like I'd been anticipating his arrival all day—I should have started a pot roast. He grabbed a beer. He loosened his tie. He ripped off his work ID tag. He sat next to me. He told me about his bad day.

"Oh, I'm sorry," I said, rubbing his shoulder. "It will be better tomorrow. Don't worry."

We went to dinner. We had wine. We smiled. We came home. We watched Anthony Bourdain's cooking travels. I never watched that, but I watched anyway.

We kissed.

PLAYING HOUSE

I didn't sleep on the sofa.

I got to touch his bald spot.

Cliff didn't pressure me for sex. He was a nice guy. Why do I call a guy "nice" if he doesn't go for sex? Does wanting sex, something natural and healthy, make a guy "bad"? Why do I always like the "bad" guys who I have to say no to?

I had to leave at four a.m. to go to the airport. It was four a.m.

"Why does this always happen?" Cliff asked. "Why is it that when I finally meet a girl, we have to part?"

"Maybe you like them *because* you are about to part," I said.

PROTOTYPE PUSSY

I got a very good look at the waiting room, better than I would have liked, because Dr. Matlock didn't show up until nine a.m. for our 6:30 a.m. interview at the Sunset Boulevard Laser Vaginal Rejuvenation Institute. The institute was clearly vulva-friendly—pink marble tile, white sofas, a view of Los Angeles from the base of Beverly Hills, palm fronds emoting tropical-vacation vibes in the corner, and the waiting room television fixed on the gossip channel E!

Dr. Matlock could turn any vulva into a perfect pussy. I didn't know there was such a thing as a prototype pussy. I wanted to know what one looked like—maybe I'd want one—so I managed to make an appointment with him before driving down to my parents' home in San Diego, with a sleepover at my grandparents' along the way.

While I waited, I read the articles reviewing Dr. Matlock's procedure. The articles were clipped from popular women's magazines and framed all proudly like graduate degrees on Dr. Matlock's office walls. Some highlights: "Are you a labia loser?" "Desire a designer vagina?" "Lisa said her boyfriend called her a bucket." Then I sat and watched the Laci Peterson story on E!, which was a downer—a domestic vulva murder.

By the time I had begun memorizing the contours of Matlock's receptionists' breasts—a three o'clock shadow from those man-made mammaries seemed like it could have shaded a picnic area for four from direct sunlight—Matlock finally arrived. He had style. The suave entry gave him a confidence that I couldn't assail despite my long wait. Firm handshake. "I've worked on the wives of kings, presidents, and executives," he said, his self-promotion as smooth as his gait.

He had a few wrinkles around his eyes—more crow's legs than feet—which showed his age, but he seemed to be a bottomless well of energy. I was constantly looking up to find he'd disappeared. He whipped out a leather-bound book that prospective clients used— much like the ones you'd find in salons, showing the various styles a hairdresser can produce—filled with before and after photos of vulvas, as well as crotch shots of playboy centerfolds.

"So a perfect pussy exists?" I asked.

"Oh, sure," he said, pointing to a photo of a bald vulva between the thighs of a supermodel. I was conflicted—did I hate the idea of a prototype pussy, or had I finally figured out what I wanted to ask my parents to get me for Chanukah?

"What women don't want is flattened or saggy labia majora," he explained, tracing vulva curves with the tip of his pen. "What they don't want is the labia minora projecting beyond the labia majora."

Zola wouldn't agree with that comment. She told me she had that vulva variation, which in some circles is known as an "overstuffed taco" or a "full-blown rose." She proudly called herself "hung," like a guy with a big cock.

"They don't want excess skin around the clitoris," Matlock continued. "What they don't want is a fat mons pubis. What they don't want is asymmetrical labia minora."

"What do they want?" I asked.

"They want the skin of the clitoris to hug it as if a piece of paper is draped tightly over an eraser," he said. "That's what they want. That's what everyone wants."

He slammed the book shut. His first appointment was already under way. He asked if we could continue the interview while he was in the procedure room.

His assistant tossed me scrubs and a mask. I changed in the bathroom.

Dr. Matlock had developed Laser Vaginal Rejuvenation (LVR) and Designer Laser Vaginoplasty (DLV) twelve years ago—the surgery was copyrighted and the moves all trademarked. LVR tightened a vagina and was often used by women who felt loose after delivering children. Matlock said the surgery enhanced sexual gratification because sexual gratification was directly related to the amount of friction the vagina could generate, but he said he couldn't fix any sexual dysfunctions. To the chagrin of many sexologists, he did not believe in Kegels to tighten or help with incontinence. "Kegels, that's a big myth," he said. "Kegels don't work."

Women could choose their preferred level of tightness by giving him an age. "Women throughout the world say, 'I want to be sixteen again, I want to be eighteen,'" he explained. "I can do that for them."

I scuttled around the surgical room. Matlock wore a sleek skullcap instead of the puffy shower cap thing everyone else wore. I hadn't eaten yet. That was a good thing. Blue crepe paper covered the operating table. There was only one small square cutout, out of which popped a cooter—a completely shaven cooter. Betty would have called the cooter a Baroque—dangling folds with switchbacks, voluminous labia minora, brownish meshing into a mauve, elaborate drapery appropriate for the window fixtures at a seventeenth-century ball. Matlock did a "before" photo shoot, the assistant snapping the shots while he took one labium per hand. He danced with them. Twist. *Click.* Spread. *Click.* To the side. *Click.* Do-si-do. *Click.*

Matlock must have been very proud of his vulva sculpting because I couldn't believe he let me inside the operating room. Through a side slit in the blue crepe paper gown, I could see a woman covered in purple markings—circles over her stomach and sides. He told me the patient was forty-one years old and would also be liposuctioned for the low "Wonderwoman" price of $15,000. I suppose that wasn't too bad for a new model vulva to drive around town.

The patient's chest rhythmically heaved in tandem with the anesthesia equipment's beep. Matlock sat in front of the cooter, confidently wielding his laser like a welder would his blowtorch. The cooter on the table had ordered a majora tightening, a minora hacking—she'd have none of that overstuffed taco—and she wanted her clit to peek out like a pencil eraser wrapped in a paper sheet. He said none of the surgeries were his own brainchild; they came from listening to women's needs. "I have concern for the woman," he said. "I consider myself a feminist. I'm here for the woman."

As Matlock cauterized a fresh cut to the perineum, the smell of burnt flesh wafted up my nose.

If Betty were in the room, I suspected she'd have handcuffed herself to this woman's remaining vulvar structures like a Greenpeace member would to a thousand-year-old sequoia facing down a chainsaw. At that moment, a profound love for the cooter welled up in me. When I saw it in a state of adversity, at its most vulnerable, I began to understand its natural beauty.

Then there was a sound I thought I recognized. Sure enough, the woman had involuntarily farted in Matlock's face as he dug into the clitoral hood, aiming to make it as thin as this page. I took the gases as an expression of displeasure by the patient's unconscious primal self. Matlock didn't flinch. He must have been accustomed to asses telling him to cease and desist.

He didn't much like detractors. When I asked him what he thought about sex therapists who disagreed with his work, he got testy and raised his voice far above the laser's droning.

"They don't know what they are talking about," he said. "I can do what they do, but they can't do what I do. They don't know surgery, yet they want to talk about it."

Matlock spread the minora and stapled them to pieces of gauze like an adolescent boy would fasten a butterfly to a bulletin board. He shaved off half their wingspan with the laser; the remnants looked like two blackened worms. As he dropped the grubs in a jar for pathology, he reiterated his goal: "Our mission is to empower women with knowledge, choice, and alternatives," he said. "It's not for everybody."

The G-shot was another alternative. For $1,850, he injected 1.5cc of collagen into the G-spot. The injection, he said, augmented the spot's size, resulting in enhanced sexual arousal and gratification for up to four months. He'd give a double dose for $2,500. "Then what happens?" I asked.

"Double the pleasure," he smirked.

After two hours, the vulva was half its original size. Matlock stitched it up; it was embroidered in red. "After" photos: *click click click*. No longer were they dramatic baroque curtains; with all the new hemlines, they were more like a doily stained with cranberry juice.

PROTOTYPE PUSSY

Clitty Rose and I hopped in the car. We charged out of Los Angeles as fast as we could. With traffic, that meant we were chugging along at about the same pace as a cud-chewing cow wandering a hayfield—that is to say, not very fast at all—but the most important thing was, we were getting away with our bat wings intact.

TIT FOR TAT

About two hours later, I pulled into my grandparents' driveway. They live in a retirement community. Every time I'm there, I feel as if I were drugged and stuck in a bad trip of circular seeing, where the same two-story house haunts my vision after every couple of tire rotations. The houses are such clones that I've had to memorize how to find their home: it's on the right side of the fifth driveway after the first right turn after the first left turn after the gate equipped with security guards who I'm pretty sure get paid to do nothing but make going anywhere a slower process.

I parked my car and knocked on their door. "Oh, sweetie," said my grandma. My grandma, Estelle, is eighty-four. There are two kinds of older ladies: the kind who grow sallow, skin going slack, revealing the details of each facial structural gap, and then there's the kind my grandma epitomizes, whose vibrancy is still visible in her ample cheeks. My grandfather, Hal, at eighty-six, shuffles as he walks—if he had mops under his shoes, the kitchen floor would sparkle—but he still goes to the gym every day and reads the paper from front to back.

They hugged me. They've been married for sixty-four years and are never apart. You can't even talk to just one of them on the phone. They don't come that way. They're Estold, they're Hartelle, and they both have to be on the line at once.

These were my father's parents I was visiting. My father said "sex" wasn't a word he ever heard growing up. His upbringing was sterile. If they had any meaty conversations, it was about whether or not the meatloaf was dry. He said that as a child, he knew about sperm and eggs but had no idea how they met up. He hypothesized that the sperm walked out of the penis, took a jaunt down the leg, then trekked up the woman's leg until it got to the uterus, at which point it shook hands with the egg, and if they got along and weren't too tired from the journey, they'd choose to make an embryo. My dad always said he didn't want me and my brothers growing up dumb like that, so he saw to it that "sex" was a word in our home.

I'd been trying to get my grandparents to agree to an interview about sex for months, but they kept turning me down. I wanted to tap wisdom from an older generation, see how far orgasms went back in the family tree, and comprehend how my father—a man who will send a *Playboy* subscription to a recently brokenhearted cousin—came forth from a gene pool of such frigidity.

My parents weren't surprised that my grandparents repeatedly declined. They didn't think I'd learn much anyway. Except for my father and his two siblings, there was no evidence my grandparents ever actually got horizontal together; their bed, ever since I could remember, was always made up—with no wrinkles—exactly like the do-not-touch-please models at Bed, Bath & Beyond. I imagined they both just stayed up all night playing Connect Four or Go

Fish and if they had to sleep, they'd do it under a lamp on a sofa chair with a magazine slipping off their laps.

But I wouldn't take no for an answer. There had to be something they could impart to me. After all, my grandfather had started sculpting naked ladies in the past ten years. Some people might say his nudie sculptures are evidence of his faculties unfastening. Really old people, really young people, and crazies (also the mentally retarded) are forgiven for faulty faculties; they get to say and do things they wouldn't be allowed to if they were like the rest of us. But if my grandpa's faculties really were slipping, I thought he should let them go some more. He's good without faculties. He enrolls each year at nearby community colleges and molds lumps of clay into the busts and behinds of live models. Now he has a harem; nude statues sit on just about every piece of my grandparents' shelving. I'm one of his biggest fans; I have three of his nudes in my bedroom: one sitting, one lying down, and one bronzed dancer named Nicole with a navel modeled after my grandmother's.

Their contradictions were confounding. But I get contradictions. I have plenty of my own—the wind-up plastic penis I like to scare company with and the naked man necklace charm I wear around my neck don't exactly jibe with my inhibited side—but I couldn't reconcile nudity in every nook and cranny with my grandparents' supposed prudery. I wanted to find out the truth.

After many attempts and light prodding, I finally figured out how to get them to share with me. I told them they could stuff me with as much food as they wanted for an eighteen-hour period—a Jewish grandmother's dream come true—if in return I got a short question-and-answer period.

I had to leave the following afternoon, but at the moment it was dinnertime. My grandma got started right away. She brought out a five-course meal—baked fish, eggplant parmesan, corn soufflé, leftover stuffed cabbage, and salad—and then my grandpa brought out a gallon of ice cream for dessert. I did my best, but I was still a little woozy from the vulva hacking I'd observed earlier in the day. In the morning they took me to IHOP—pancakes, omelets, and oatmeal. Two hours later we went out to lunch at a Mexican joint— fajitas, ceviche, and shrimp tostada. My gastrointestinal system was freaking out. But it would be worth it, I told myself.

When we returned from our eating escapades, a bronze nude ballerina doing an arabesque greeted us in the foyer. My grandparents settled in the study.

"Okay," said my grandpa. "We're ready."

I sat down across from them. I didn't feel bad about making them do this, not anymore at least; I'd earned this. But I wanted to go into it slowly. I didn't want to freak them out. I saw a bandage on my grandpa's arm.

"You're all bruised," I said, breaking the ice.

"Yeah, my skin's thinner," he said. "I have to carry Band-Aids in my wallet now."

"He used to carry around a different kind of protection," my grandma said.

They both looked at each other and chortled.

If I wasn't mistaken, my grandparents had just made an allusion to prophylactics. I took a second to recalibrate.

"How'd you feel when my dad got into sex therapy?" I asked. "Did that make you uncomfortable?"

"He did a lot of nice work," said my grandma. "Acorn doesn't fall so far from the tree," she continued, looking at me as if I might be some sort of smooth oval nut.

"We're proud of your father," said Grandpa.

"We went to one of his classes," my grandma said. "I thought that generation of student—you know, the sixties—was much freer, much different from our generation. I felt they went in knowing a lot about sex and life in general, but they really didn't because the questions they asked, they were real novices, they didn't know anything!"

My grandpa began telling me about the beginnings of their relationship. After only thirty dates, he said he wooed my grandmother by telling her that if he died in the war—this was during World War II—she'd get a ten-thousand-dollar stipend without ever having to live with him.

"That was nothing to sneeze at," he said, laughing.

My grandma accepted the proposal; she got married a virgin and used all the money she had saved to buy a fur coat on their Miami honeymoon. She said when she was younger, it was really simple: the only thing she had to know about sex was that she wasn't supposed to have any. No masturbation either. "It was real chaste," she said. There were no expectations to live up to because no one knew what to expect.

"This is getting kind of more personal," I said, still treading lightly. "You can tell me if you don't want to answer. But how did you know about the female orgasm?"

"How did I know?" my grandma said. "Because I experienced it!"

"Did you ever get any advice or anything?"

"No," she said. "Well, actually I was getting married and my gynecologist said just one sentence. He said, 'Anything goes in the bedroom,' and I remembered it."

"Has it helped you?"

"Yeah," she said. "It's good advice. It gave permission to do whatever he wanted to do."

"Wait a minute," my grandpa said. "Whatever *you* wanted to do. You just said whatever *he* wanted to do. There's a duality here."

TIT FOR TAT

"Well, you know what I mean," she said. "Anything goes between the couple."

"'Cause you said anything *he* wanted to do," my grandpa repeated.

"Well, I was just giving a little aside," she said.

"Were you immediately orgasmic?" I asked, breaking it up.

"Yeah," said Grandma.

"Oh, yeah," said Grandpa.

"Yeah," she said.

"Very," he said.

"On the first night," I said, a bit dumbfounded. "Really?"

"Not the first night," he said. "The first night there was a problem. She was all sealed up."

"Yes, a very thick seal," said my grandma.

"Then the second night? How was that?"

My grandma blushed and rubbed her palms against her thighs. Her white Reeboks tapped the floor. "It was good," she said. "I enjoyed it."

"You want to say anything more?"

My grandpa chimed in, "Well, we usually had the orgasm together," he said. "We liked it best that way."

Okay . . . umm . . . so I guess orgasms went back at least two generations. No debate about that, apparently. They were spilling it so easily. They duped me. They just acted shy so they could cram food down my throat, obviously.

My grandma cleared her throat. "Why aren't you writing a *Gone With the Wind*–type book? Wouldn't that be nice?"

"Our present sex life is *Gone With the Wind*," Grandpa said. They both laughed.

He suddenly got very serious. Then he told me about his erectile dysfunction. "Have you heard of that?" he said. "I wish

I didn't have this erectile dysfunction thing, but I do, so there you go."

My grandpa said it'd been fifteen years since they had had sex.

"Hon, no, it was ten years ago," my grandma said, correcting him. "I remember. I remember it well."

Maybe all my grandfather's unrealized sexual energies went into the statues peeking out from every corner.

My grandpa got up to get a drink. As he ambled away, I leaned toward my grandma.

"Do you still have orgasms?"

"If I wanted to, I would," she said, "but I don't want to."

"Why not?" I asked.

"'Cause I like to do it with Grandpa. We're like this," she said, clasping her hands together. "Maybe it's not so good . . . but . . ."

My grandpa walked up to her, breaking off our conversation, and offered a diet ice tea. "Here, hon," he said. "Drink it."

She tipped it toward her lips, took a couple sips. I heard it gurgle down her throat, and then she handed it back. He brought it back to his seat and sat down.

"Sex isn't everything," Grandpa began.

"Orgasm isn't the only important thing. It's only one facet," said Grandma.

I felt a little jab. Maybe this was their way of telling me I was looking for the wrong thing.

"Age does things to your body and needs," they agreed. "It changes. We hug a lot."

"What do you find to be the most important thing, then?" I asked.

"It's love and respect," my grandma said.

"It's responding to one another's needs," my grandpa said.

"I rub his back with lotion," said Grandma.

"I help you put your bra on," said Grandpa, looking at my grandma.

"You snap it on because I can't," she said, looking at him.

My grandpa leaned forward, the light moving off his face. In a monotone, he said, "I call that tit for tat."

FROSTED FLAKES

When I arrived in San Diego, Keena wasn't home yet. They were still working at the nursery. Looking at their bookshelves, which I'd scanned hundreds of times for some good reading material, I began to recognize books I'd never noticed before. They were the ones I'd recently bought and stacked on my own shelves. Next to my father's old bound thesis—*The Study of Sexual Attitude Reassessment*—which I knew existed but had never touched, let alone read, there were the Kinsey Reports, books by Masters and Johnson, *The Hite Report*, and even *The Joy of Sex*. Our libraries had become freakily similar.

Over the next week at home, I planned to help my parents prepare for the forty-three guests we had coming over for Thanksgiving dinner but also to confront them about how they raised me. I wanted answers about how I'd wound up like this.

At least one thing I could be grateful for was that I now knew there was plenty of orgasm in my genes. If I straightened all this stuff out, I'd be coming all the time: it was in my DNA.

When my parents finished work, we went out to Chinese food. I regaled them with stories of Dr. Matlock, whom I'd come to call the Box Cutter; of Ray Noonan; and for the finale, I gave them the truth about the Altman grandparents.

"They're superorgasmic," I said. "Simultaneous was their norm!"

My parents' mouths dropped open. My dad dropped his chopsticks. He'd probably thought all this time that he was being rebellious in his sexiness, but it turns out he had just blossomed conventionally from the planted seed.

"I don't believe it," said my mom. "I never would have thought."

"Why did they say they never talked about it, then?" asked my dad.

"They asked if I'd heard of the 'don't ask, don't tell' policy," I said.

My dad shook his head as he ate a sweet and sour shrimp.

"They said it never came up," I continued, shrugging.

I'd never seen my dad look like that before. "That's like saying it just happened to come up in our household," he said.

My mom said if I had asked her parents when they were still alive, they would have avoided my questions in the same way they did hers when she was growing up—by sneaking nonchalantly into the other room to watch their Dobermans run in circles, leaving piddle stains in concentric streams.

As I finished recalling a few more choice tidbits from the interview, we all scraped the final bites off our plates. I expected, because my parents were so open, that they'd be ready and raring to get their stories down on my digital recorder. But for such open people, my parents didn't seem particularly inclined at the moment to share. I had never thought my grandparents would be the better interview subjects. Instead, my parents asked me if

I'd thought of publishing under a pseudonym. "How about Pig Latin?" my dad suggested, lightly laughing. "We'll be Enkay and Eenaday."

Two days later, my mom took the day off from work to spend with me, because once Thanksgiving preparations began, we wouldn't get a moment alone. Behind my parents' house, there's a rural preserve filled with craggy oaks, crackly dry brush, and granite boulders so large a bulldozer would be as useless as a plastic fork to move them. We went on a hike to catch up. The sun beat down on us as we went up the steep hills; with the incline, my mom's breathing steadily became heavier. It's an annoying sound—the labored breathing—the sound of getting older, a reminder of not lasting forever. She's just as human as my dad, who is just as human as I am, and just as human as Norman Mailer, who had died the previous week.

Earlier that morning, I'd approached my parents as they sat in their customary breakfast nook positions. (It's a round table, but it somehow seemed like my father was always situated at the head.) My brother Logan was due to arrive later in the evening from Boulder, where he was going to school, and I wanted to confront them before too many people were around. I also didn't want all these looming questions muddling my good senses as guests arrived; I'd already upset my other brother, Matt, when he'd called. I yelled into the phone by way of greeting, "Mattilingus!"

There was a silence.

"Mara, don't ever call me that again!" he demanded.

"What?"

It took me a second, but yeah, I got it: it was gross. There was only one thing I could think of that ended in *lingus,* and it certainly wasn't my brother. But that's how fixated I was on that stuff, so full of it that it seeped out inappropriately.

FROSTED FLAKES

"Sorry."

My dad was engrossed in the newspaper when I came to confront him. "Dad," I said, trying to get his attention.

Every morning it's the same routine. My dad brings two bowls—the yellow one for him and the green and white one for my mom—a big and a little spoon, and eight boxes of cereal for elaborate mixing. It's the same thing every day—I know, tedious, right?—but Keena says it doesn't get boring. Cereal is number one on my dad's food pyramid, especially Frosted Flakes, which I found ironic when I learned that the conservative Dr. John Harvey Kellogg had originally developed Cornflakes in the nineteenth century because he believed bland foods would dampen people's—and especially women's—"inappropriate" passions and sex drive. It'd really get that Kellogg now to see his flakes glazed with sugar, not to mention being slurped down by an openly passionate couple.

My dad blended his cereals as my mom bobbed her tea bag in and out of hot water. I was there. They were there. I had my recorder. I could ask them anything.

"Why did you tell me it was black?" I said.

What the fuck was that? That's what came out. The question just puddled up in my throat and I yakked it out.

"What was black?" asked my dad.

"Black, nothingness," I said. "You know, when I die."

He folded his paper and stilled his spoon.

"Was that a bad answer?" he asked.

"I think it scarred me," I said.

"You go up to heaven," he said, smiling. "Is that better?"

I rolled my eyes.

"It's too late," I said. "You already ruined it."

"I couldn't tell you something I didn't believe," he said. "Death is something we have to reconcile or deny. You choose."

They sensed I wasn't satisfied, but even I didn't know what I wanted them to say.

He laughed. "It's funny, the things people remember," he said, and went back to slurping his Frosted Flakes–sweetened milk.

My mom and I zigzagged along the trail. I was already feeling stifled at home. I felt like I wasn't being productive. My mom says it's good to rest sometimes, but resting felt like a waste of time. I wanted to see execution, production, realization, markers of progress. How else do you prove to yourself you exist?

We talked as I pulled brambles out of the path. I brought up the orgasmic journey.

"What are yours like?" I asked.

As she sucked in some water, she told me that orgasm was a very intimate thing. She said that she was still figuring it out.

"It's one thing to have a sex-positive household," she said. "One's own sex life is a completely different matter. It's not always easy for me, either. There are still frontiers in front of me. The layers keep peeling off."

This was a weird feeling. I had no idea what she was talking about. Who were these people, my parents? If they were going to play this game of not knowing everything, they should have started a long time ago. In one minute, she was somehow managing to shatter the image of her that I'd steadily developed for the past 13,665,600 minutes of my life.

We stopped at a ledge with a view over the valley.

"You know, Mara," my mom said, as she looked out at the horizon, "you used to touch yourself when you were a little girl. I just wanted you to know that."

FROSTED FLAKES

"Oh," I said, my cheeks flushing. "Really?" I turned away from her. "Look at that," I said, pointing at the mountaintops. "A lot of construction going on out here, huh?"

"We are who we are before we know who we are," she said.

I turned back around to face her. I stared for a second. She's smaller than I am by an inch. Weird that I was ever inside there— maybe I knew myself better when I was part of her.

But what the hell was she talking about? Whatever it was, it sounded smart. Smart mom-stuff to impart. But I was thankful when our conversation devolved into how many packages of turkey stuffing we should buy. It was discomfiting that she knew things about me that I didn't know. *It's funny the things people remember.* That phrase popped into my mind from the conversation I'd had earlier in the morning with my father. If that was the case, what were the things I'd forgotten?

While we went back to the house, I got to thinking more. If it was true, if I did touch myself when I was little, when did I lose touch? Do we all lose touch in some way as we get older? When I got back home, I wondered what else I had lost along the way. I took out my journals, the ones I'd recently excavated, and started foraging through the prose. I concentrated on searching for myself in old objects, letters, and locations around the house.

I'd scheduled some phone sessions with Rori before I'd left New York. When we talked, I told her about things I'd found in my journals, especially things that embarrassed me. There were emotions I didn't remember feeling and moments I'd completely blocked out; but the things I wrote, the stuff I wanted—most of it had come true, almost to a fault.

After breaking up with Evan, I'd written a promise to myself.

Now reading it, I almost upchucked at the drama I'd inflicted on myself. What a soap opera I was then. I read it to Rori:

> I am wary now and will not let my love be pulled away from me like a kite in the wind. I will hold tight to that string, very tight. I cannot hurt like that hurt. I will not do that again.

I laughed at my overwrought language, but at the same time, it made me sad. I'd listened to myself very well. I'd not only held onto the string, but I'd buried it under all my books, all my professional goals, anything big and heavy enough so that I wouldn't have to constantly worry about letting it go.

Rori told me that it seemed I'd made something as pleasurable as orgasm into a goal. "You're not allowing pleasure unless it's involved in the accomplishment of a task," she said. "What is it like to just want?"

I didn't know what I wanted; I'd become so good at sublimating my body's desires that I had to logically decide what I wanted instead of feeling it from the inside. Simple decisions caused trouble. I often couldn't even decipher if I craved a chocolate chip or peanut butter cookie—I fell back on calorie counts to aid my taste buds' selection.

When our session was over, I lay on my bed, thinking. The sun crawled toward the horizon, the evening light streaming through the bedroom window, washing everything in pinks. I looked at the purple vibrator, which was somehow actually green; I wanted to use it. I wanted to try it. I wanted to find *that* piece of me. It was there already, it had to be. But not here. Not now. Not in my old bedroom. It was glowing pink, like a baby's room. I felt not dormant but retrograde, backward, almost on rewind.

FROSTED FLAKES

FUCKED IN A WAY

THAT DOESN'T CORRELATE

The night before Thanksgiving, my brother Logan and I stayed up talking outside on the patio while Keena went for their nightly co-shower. We'd all gone grocery shopping earlier in the day. A lot of eating was going to happen. We were going to collectively add a large amount of Earth's matter to ourselves with all the imminent self-stuffing. The more territory you own, the better, isn't that how it goes? I was going to look at my impending weight gain as land acquisition.

Logan's only a year older than me. He's one of my closest friends. I've forgiven him for those years in high school when I'd wake up to find a friend of mine had disappeared, been beamed without a trace, practically *Star Trek*–style, into his bed. I popped the cork off a bottle of wine. It glug-glug-glugged into his glass. We clinked. "To our health," we said.

Logan told me that ever since he started studying Judaism, he kept noticing the number thirteen. He said that in Kabbalah, the Hebrew words for "love" (*ahava*) and "one" (*echad*) each had the numerical value of thirteen. He then explained that both words are aspects of God. I told him I kept seeing elevens everywhere and I couldn't decide if it meant I had to go to the bathroom twice for a #1 or if I should add them up and go #2 once.

Logan had gone on a free trip to Israel called Birthright about two years ago. He came back Jewish, but not the Jewish I am. He came back the real kind of Jewish—no shellfish or pork, no light switches or phones on Sabbath, not even any goy pussy anymore. He kept saying I should go to Israel. If I did, he said, I would understand where I came from; I would look around and realize: *These are my people*. That's what happened to him; he looked around at the people cutting in line, being pushy, and saying exactly what was on their mind, and he was like: *These are my people*. So I did what he told me: I signed up for the trip. I figured at the least I'd get to investigate my orgasmic ancestral roots. I was scheduled to go in January, less than two months away. We decided to hold off on the Jew talk until I could relate, and instead we related about how our parents had fucked us up.

As I poured the last drop of wine into Logan's tumbler, he explained how he felt about our upbringing. He thought all the sex talk growing up made him too comfortable with the subject matter and screwed up his boundaries—too permeable. Meanwhile, he said, he had girlfriend after girlfriend whom he dumped because none of them lived up to the ultimate Altman relationship model. As we uncorked the next bottle, we had an unfortunate epiphany: we realized we weren't fucked up in the same way.

"I never have relationships," I said.

"I have too many relationships," he said.

"I'm unfucked," I said. "I don't fuck enough."

"I fuck too much," he said. "I'm overly fucked."

"What the fuck?" I said.

FUCKED IN A WAY THAT DOESN'T CORRELATE

We were oppositely fucked.

Didn't the fact that we were opposite invalidate our upbringing as a correlating factor? What fucks us up? Does just being in the world do shit to us? I asked Logan why God doesn't talk to us anymore. A couple thousand years ago there were burning bushes, parting seas, rules engraved on stone tablets proclaiming God's will, telling everyone what they needed to know.

"God even freaking talked into stone tablets," I said. "He somehow typed shit into stone. You'd think he could just pick up the phone or something."

Why did God suddenly go silent? We could use a little advice here, I said, a little direction, please. Logan stared on. Maybe he was translating the alcohol percentage of our wine into Kabbalistic significance. I looked at the label. The percentage was thirteen.

"God, was it you?" I said. "Did you fuck us up?"

It was obviously time for bed.

ACORN

The next morning, I was totally fresh, totally in the mood for my yearly brawl with poultry carcass. My dad and I challenge each other to cram as much stuffing as possible inside the turkeys' cavities because we don't believe in stuffing that isn't actually stuffed—it's actually just breadcrumbs until it's stuffed.

We had two turkeys. My dad was in charge of the free range; I had the conventional. We dug out the giblets, tossed them aside. Then there's the turkey neck all up inside there. I reached up to my elbow into the carcass's hollow. I felt it—long, sinewy, and cold. I gauged its firmness: quite taut. I pulled it out. The turkey neck never looked quite like it did at that moment: I swear it was the turkey's penis. Turkey is uncomplicated like men, I discovered. I felt embarrassed as I yanked it free. It was lewd, crass, insensitive, and extremely rigid. All those unanswered questions were definitely screwing with my reality. They were making me sick, perverted. I hid the turkey dick behind my back so my parents wouldn't see; I tossed it, nonchalantly, into the trash can. Then my dad extracted his turkey neck. It slumped over. He was putting it aside so he could wash the carcass, but I couldn't help myself. I couldn't shut myself up. "Rough year, huh?" I said, referring to his drooping member. I said I must be losing my faculties.

My mom was there and she laughed. My dad laughed, too. Of course they did; they were the ones who had taught me to be like that. They must have birthed me in the gutter.

We finished triumphantly, with both turkeys in the oven.

Then I went solicitation-crazy. I wallpapered the house with flyers. My parents let me. I pasted the papers everywhere, by the hors d'oeuvre table and the pool table and the dinner table, in the kitchen and the living room.

The flyers informed the guests of my current quest and asked them to please write any orgasm information—anonymously, if they'd like—on an index card and insert it into the Kleenex box that I'd transformed, by way of magic markers and construction paper, into the Orgasm Box.

The dinner was a success. The turkey butt, which is my grandma's favorite part—she says it's the most flavorful—was even efficiently transported to her plate. She always thinks someone is going to steal it.

Grandma, when you're with us, we'll be sure you get ass.

After everyone left, I emptied out my Orgasm Box. Three cards fell out. I kept shaking the box, banging on the bottom, but nothing else came out. Only three cards? Only one in every 14.3 Americans has something to say about orgasm?

That was a let-down. I blamed the low response rate on the tryptophan.

The following day, after cleanup, it was finally time to face my parents. It had to be then; I was leaving for San Francisco the next day. But none of us seemed particularly inclined to have the conversation. It made sense; as soon as I wanted to know about it all, they withheld. But when I didn't want to know, like during the impressionable part of my life, when I was prone to scarring, they were like broken faucets with their information—they couldn't keep it from pouring out.

They both sat on the sofa in the living room. My mom had her feet up, her arms wrapped around her legs. My dad leaned into the cushion and rubbed his bald head. If he had added some carnauba wax to that motion, I could have easily used the polished surface as a mirror to pluck my eyebrows in. I sat across from them. When I peered at my dad's face, the part of his thick glasses that stuck away from his temples caught my attention. The scene behind him blurred into gobbledygook. My looking at him looking at me looked like an oil spill—everything was the same.

"Okay, shoot," said my dad.

So I began, reluctantly.

"How are we—I am speaking for my brothers, too—supposed to live up to your relationship?" I said. "You've set impossible standards."

"Don't put us up on a pedestal," my dad said. "Just because we don't do it in front of you doesn't mean we don't have arguments."

"Yeah," my mom said. "We have arguments."

"We have arguments," Keena said.

This was going nowhere.

So I went to topic two: I asked why they were so open with us, why we had lived in a mininudist colony, why sexuality was so much a part of our growing up.

"We wanted you to be comfortable about your bodies," my mom said, "and never have it be a surprise how babies were made."

"We hoped that love and sex would be natural and not so extremely capitalized," said my dad. "No capital letters or quotation marks, just that it's a part of life and easy for you."

"But how'd you get comfortable enough to study sex if it was a taboo subject in your house?" I asked. "You said Grandma and Grandpa didn't talk about it at all."

"What can be more interesting to think about or talk about than sex?" my dad answered. "Especially if you were kind of inhibited, like me. As you grow up you work on what's hardest for you, hopefully."

He said he focused his thesis on sexuality for a reason: so he could desensitize himself.

"You were inhibited?" I said. "Really?"

I looked to my mom for confirmation. "Mom, really?"

Here was a mind-fuck. I knew that my dad studied sex therapy, but I'd always assumed it was because he was so comfortable sexually that he could spread his comfort to the masses of frigid souls, not because he needed four years of post-grad work to figure out his own hang-ups.

My mom nodded. "You're doing more or less the same thing Ken did to get comfortable," she said. They smiled at each other knowingly and then looked at me like I was an acorn next to its tree.

I had come looking for orgasm in my heredity; instead I'd found the origination of my DNA receptors that clicked on inhibition and prudery. I'd thought all this time that I was being rebellious in my unsexiness, but it turned out that I had just blossomed conventionally from the planted seed.

And what would this revelation have been without the chorus to my life?

"You're a late bloomer," my dad said, "like me."

He was smiling pretty big by this point, my dad. Like father, like daughter. I was feeling disoriented. Just like the Altmans to throw in a twist like that. I couldn't muster another question. I didn't have one. My dad told me that if I was interested, I could take his dissertation with me and read about his journey.

"Just don't lose it," he said. "There's only one."

I excused myself to pack up my stuff for my early morning flight. Then I pulled my father's large rectangular thesis off the shelf to bring to bed and started reading. I'd always thought it'd be full of such interesting and vivid stuff—so vivid that I'd always chosen the safe route and avoided it—but in one minute, all my dad's desensitization put me right to sleep.

FEELING FORSAKEN IN THE CLIT OF THE COUNTRY (AND THE BURNING BUSH)

After three days at my cousin's place in San Francisco, I was completely exhausted. My cousin has a one-year-old daughter. Courageous, the choice to procreate. The toddler likes to scream from two to four in the morning, every morning. It's a siren, the bleating, blinking kind. Its skin flashes as it wails. Little foam earplugs, purple, on day two saved me from a sleep-deprived half-conscious attempt to tie my tubes.

But this kid was interesting. She might have been the me my mom told me I used to be. She humped objects with a diaper on, she stripped every chance she got, she manipulated dolls obscenely in public, and she poked around in her crotch with flagrant abandon. If perpetrated by an adult, these actions would have put her in lockup. The slammer. Incarcerated. No questions asked. I admired her for that; she was taking advantage while she could. This chick was truly in touch. This chick, she had clarity.

I could have used some clarity after a couple days in San Francisco: so far it hadn't exactly gone according to plan. On top of that, I'd just found out Rafiq was getting married, another friend had eloped, and stupid Facebook kept updating me on everyone from high school who posted photos of themselves with boyfriends or armloads of newly arrived genetic material. Even my prostitute-loving, go-go-bar-frequenting friend in Bangkok changed his status to "in a relationship." I was feeling bad at being human. I wondered if the circuitry for my biological clock was actually cross-wired with my ability to come. Trip one and, like the domino effect, it'd trip the other?

My aunt, who also lived in San Francisco, saved the day. She told me I could stay at her place until she was sick of me. She liked her space. I got it: I liked my space too. But finally, I had some solitude.

She's got this whole two-bedroom place to herself. She's an ob-gyn; I used to want to be an ob-gyn when I was little because I thought the apartment came with her title. She gets to see it all from her Telegraph Hill view: the Bay Bridge, Alcatraz, Treasure Island, the teeny-weeny people way down by the ferry building. But then when I was ten she brought me into the delivery room. I got to see what being an ob-gyn really meant. Something the size of a watermelon charging through the middle of a bagel: tell me, how is that a good idea?

I didn't want to be an ob-gyn anymore, but that didn't stop me from admiring my aunt. She's been married twice and twice divorced. She's a fulfilled woman—not an ounce of spinster to her—who doesn't need a wedding band to tell her she's whole. She loves my parents but talks about their interdependence almost like it's a sickness. "I wouldn't want what they've got," she always says. I get her, I know what she's talking about, and even though I agree, there's a twinge of me that sometimes suspects it's jealousy. (I think Rori would say I'm projecting.)

FEELING FORSAKEN IN THE CLIT OF THE COUNTRY

Unfortunately, my aunt just didn't quite get *me*, or at least my current undertaking.

"I don't understand why you're doing this, Mara," she said. "You should have just told me about the orgasm; I would have taken you to a shop, we'd get you a vibrator, and it'd be done with already."

On a certain level, I agreed with my aunt. I understood her bit of vexation; I was a little annoyed with myself too, not to mention sexually frustrated. I'd been stringing myself along, acting like one big tease to my own body. I couldn't wait to experience what I'd heard people talk about for so long, and meanwhile I conjectured that it couldn't be much further than one battery's worth of vibrations away, so I wasn't exactly sure what was stopping me. Maybe so much hinged upon experiencing my orgasm that by that point I'd almost psyched myself out. What if the incident didn't answer all the questions I'd hoped it would? If I didn't try, I didn't have to be let down yet.

"Just don't spend too much time on it," she said, slipping out the door for work. "It's getting boring."

I had such high hopes for the clit of the country, but things were moving really slowly. I'd contacted Joseph Kramer, a well-known sexological body worker in the area. Sexological body workers are erotic educators; their lessons are often hands-on. He refused to talk to me, explaining that sex writers quashed people's sexual creativity. He signed off with this, a Wilhelm Reich quote: "Those who are psychically ill need but one thing—complete and repeated genital gratification."

So then I called Satya, Zola's *dakini* friend. I knew some of Zola's work had to do with, um, genital stimulation, but I wasn't sure what Satya was offering. I wanted to make an appointment to find out. Would it be awkward if a female stranger gave me my first orgasm? Would that mean anything? In her sultry voice, she talked slowly and rhythmically. I kept interrupting her, but not on purpose; the dimension I lived in just seemed to go about three times faster than hers. I felt like the annoying automatic toilet function that flushes before your business is done. But we finally managed to agree on a date and time. She only had one slot that worked; it was the day before I had to leave.

Dorrie Lane, the Oakland-based inventor of vulva puppets, had yet to get back to me with a time when she could meet. I was thinking she could teach me how to manipulate those puffy stuffed-minora lips correctly because, you know, it's not like Picchu, my supposed mascot, had really spoken up that much.

Then there was the call with Dr. Annie Sprinkle, a former porn star. What she is now is hard to sum up. She sometimes uses the title Post-Porn Modernist. She has her Ph.D. in human sexuality, does performance art, writes, teaches, and directs her own videos. Out of everyone, I was most excited to speak to her face-to-face. This was the woman who has had sex with 3,500 people in ten years. She might have been the most orgasmic woman I'd ever heard of. We'd been planning to meet after keeping in touch during the preceding months. But when I called her, it went something like this:

Me: It's Mara. How's it going?

Annie: Mia!

Me: Actually, it's Mara.

Annie: Who?

Me: Mara, the writer.

Annie: You're not Mia?

Me: I'm Mara. The no-orgasm girl, remember?

Annie: Oh, I see, yeah . . . I thought you were someone else.

She had that tone in her voice like vegetarians do when you tell them you eat meat.

FEELING FORSAKEN IN THE CLIT OF THE COUNTRY

She didn't have time to interview anymore. She had a gallery exhibition opening on Saturday and was running late. "Why don't you just stop by on Friday while we're setting up?" she said. It didn't sound promising.

Since it was only Wednesday at this time, I stopped by One-Taste headquarters, hoping to run into The Gasm to get some insight into the MEANING OF ORGASM.

Once I stepped into the OneTaste foyer, I felt discombobulated, though that's how I always felt around those people. I'd been back to OneTaste's other branch in New York several times, but I still hadn't paid the fee to take off my trousers. I felt disjointed, like I was watching a movie that was supposed to be seen with those 3-D glasses, but I had forgotten my glasses, so I was the only one seeing blurry images up on the screen. Maybe when I got my orgasm I'd see clearly. That's what I kept telling myself anyway.

They all live together—beds in the same room. They romp in front of one another. They are investigating sensation, they say. Like how a friend of mine and his girlfriend screw other people in front of each other to explore jealousy. They call each other research partners and do fieldwork. I like science, but I haven't gotten my head around this method quite yet.

Then I spotted Nicole Daedone, The Gasm herself, in the lobby café. It was the first time I had seen her outside of YouTube. She looked taller. She had long brown hair and was wearing black high heels and stretch pants.

She had the attention of the whole room, which made her seem in many places at once. People were waiting, at a distance, to talk to her. She talked to a woman at a table; the girl had blond hair and eyes brimming with tears about to spill. The Gasm touched her chest, and the tears began to fall. She smiled serenely as the girl's body jerked.

I watched her too, but I didn't approach. I was being a pussy. I wondered how many cocks The Gasm had touched and, if placed head to scrotum, would the lineup be long enough to stretch to Nevada? That's power, an interstate penis path. My personal penis path would only reach a few steps away, barely to where her assistant, Alisha, was standing.

I thought I might as well go through protocol since I was too intimidated to ask The Gasm for an interview myself. I traversed my penis path and asked Alisha for an appointment. "Nicole's busy," she answered.

So I guess my subconscious made The Gasm available because that night I dreamed that I met her. I didn't have to ask her anything. In my dream, she touched my sternum just like she did the woman who was crying at the table. She said, "You know why God hasn't spoken in quite some time? It's because everyone's been looking for the wrong burning bushes. It has nothing to do with shrubbery," she said, pointing toward her crotch. "Darling, it's this burning bush that God talks through."

When I awoke, I heard a rattle and I suspected that my brain had come loose, but upon closer inspection it was just the cling-clanging of my long, dangly earrings; I'd forgotten to take them off.

I looked down at my bush—nothing was talking or flaming, but I did wonder if that's why my brother had a thing for redheads lately—and was surprised. It only took San Francisco three days to make me go nuts.

If I went nuts, like really nuts, or say I lost my mind to something like Alzheimer's disease, I wondered who would take me on walks, but even more important, who'd pluck the insurgent hairs on my tit? Maybe husbands *are* worthwhile if they're good for that.

So now, as I unpacked my stuff in my aunt's guest room, I got on the computer. I had to see if anyone had gotten back to me. No e-mails, none at all, not even from my mother. I thought maybe the Internet had died until I addressed an e-mail to myself and received it. It was a lonely feeling—me being the only one in my in-box.

When my aunt came home, she made dinner. She baked fresh salmon with lavender salt and tossed vibrant greens with a mixture of Meyer lemon and extra-virgin olive oil. I said I wasn't hungry, and then I ate everything. I told her I'd be at OneTaste again tomorrow for an interview with The Gasm's assistant. Then I told her about OneTaste—"all in a warehouse, they have sex, and . . ."

She cut me off. "That's really uninteresting to me," she said. "All these people are stuck in the sixties. Been there, done that. Really boring."

She told me to have my orgasm already so I could move on to a more interesting topic. "Don't get fixated," she said. "Boring."

Maybe she just thought that because she had her head up cooter all day, but either way, I felt like the clit of the country was rejecting me. My aunt retired to her bedroom; she had work early the next morning. I wasn't sleepy, so I cracked open my dad's thesis again. That thing worked better than a sleeping pill.

DUT DUT DUT

The following morning, I hopped in the shower. There's a window in there that faces the bay. I saw birds flitter past, and as I did, I caught sight of the detachable showerhead. I took it off as Fiona's words came to mind: There ain't nothing that works like a carefully placed water stream to the clitty. I was ready. I didn't care that no one was calling me back; this was the perfect place to have my first orgasm, in an incredibly discerning single woman's apartment with a priceless view. I was INDEPENDENT. I lay down with my back flat on the porcelain tub. I aimed the torrent, full blast, at the juncture between my legs. I was going to hose the orgasm out of me. I breathed. I squeezed, even though Barbara Carrellas, the woman who taught me the breath energy orgasm, which ended in hyperventilation, said no squeezing. *Breathe*, but I couldn't: The water was overcoming me. It ricocheted off my cooter and sprayed my eyes. My contacts dried out. They stuck uncomfortably as I tried to blink. For an instant, I was suspended, like the bridge. It felt like cold metal balls were spiraling their way down my femurs and propelling out of my toes. For some reason, I started seeing the faces of all the people in the world without access to clean water. I'd seen people in India line up for hours to fill a small bucket from a tanker truck. I'd read that women take on average anywhere from ten to twenty minutes to come; by that time, a village could fill up a small swimming pool with the runoff from my cunt. This wasn't right, but I didn't have to make a moral decision. The moment had passed. The high pressure was like a shot of Novocaine to my clit; by the end of minute one, Clitty Rose was completely numb.

I got out and dried off. As I dressed, my clit slowly sputtered back to life—first with a jag of prickles and then in and out of tingle fits. I charged myself with one account of attempted orgasm and condemned myself, once again, to better luck next time.

Before heading out the door for my OneTaste interview, I plugged my purple vibrator into an outlet. It blinked blinked blinked with life, like a little cell phone charging up.

When I arrived at OneTaste, my pussy was still having intermittent aftershocks. As I interviewed Alisha, I was distracted. I talked in rhythm to the beat of my crotch: *dut dut dut*. Whatever I said, the syllabic meter had to match.

"Though we're all fixated and wanting of the thing we don't have," she said, "we're totally confronted by it when it's there."

Yes. Yes. Yes.

"No one's talking about sex, and everyone is locking it down," she said. "It breeds social disease."

Yes. Yes. Yes.

I didn't ask what the MEANING OF ORGASM was (and I didn't give up my quest to ask The Gasm that question in person), but I gathered from our interview that, somehow, female orgasm has the potential to cure the world of all its ills.

Another good reason to have one.

SHE KNOWS A LOT ABOUT FEMALE ORGASM

The next day, there were Salvation Army Santa Clauses ringing bells along the way to the Center for Sex and Culture, where I was to meet Carol Queen. They were doing it so fervently that I was now of the belief that that kind of banging was also a form of sexual release.

I must have gotten caught up in my yuletide hypothesis, because I was soon lost. I was late for my appointment and didn't have Carol's number. I called up Annie Sprinkle to get it—all these sex people seemed to know each other—since I was supposed to meet Annie at the gallery later anyway. And after our last conversation, confirmation seemed necessary.

"It's Mara," I said.

"Mia!" she said. "How are you?"

Not this again—was I really so awful? I had to tell her that it was actually me, the anorgasmic one, again.

"Oh," she said. "I thought you were someone else."

She told me that she was sorry and still couldn't fathom making time for an interview that day. She was frazzled and late to install her show, a tribute to Marcel Duchamp. She had planned a séance for opening night, tomorrow, where she'd use a medium to channel Duchamp into the room and then make love to him with energy.

"We're going to have an energy orgasm," she said.

She said I could come by later in the afternoon and help set up, if I wanted. She said she felt bad for botching our appointment.

Carol Queen, besides being a prolific sex writer and educator, also ran the Center for Sex and Culture. Everything about her said librarian—a rubber band held her brownish-gray hair tightly away from her face; wire-rimmed glasses perched upon a delicate nose; black slacks, flat shoes, and a T-shirt that read I LOVE FEMALE OR-GASM (okay, she was a very special kind of librarian). We sat down on the two sofas; they were yellow velvet with purple embroidery, so soft and mushy that it was like descending into silly putty. My tush would surely leave an impression.

Carol had started masturbating with her father's vibrator (he was a barber and gave his clients pulsating post-clip shoulder rubs) at fifteen. She said it was so loud that it sounded like a helicopter was landing and the electrical surge would make the television roll. "If I wanted privacy, it had to be when people went grocery shopping," she said. "For many years, no one ever saw me going to the grocery store."

I got ahead of myself again when we started discussing all the different positions one could come in. Carol could come in almost any position, even standing up. She had trained herself that way. She said I had to deal with an element called proprioception, the body's ability to know where it is even when the eyes are closed— you know if you're sitting down or standing up. "Proprioception has an erotic component," she said. "If you learned to have orgasms on your back and then you get on top, it might be harder to have an orgasm." She said it takes a lot of practice and training, but people can have an orgasm in any position if they want to.

I wasn't sure what I wanted from her, but I came out of our meeting inspired about prospective coming positions—while in handstand, hula-hooping, sitting at a boring lecture, in Revolving Half Lotus yoga pose. The only negative was looking down at the imprint my ass had made on the couch, which was wider than I would have liked.

I went to the Femina Potens gallery straightaway. Nothing was set up. Only a single volunteer was there, repainting the walls white. She hadn't met Annie before, either. Piles of suitcases lay on the floor; around them were sprawled feathers, mannequins, sequins, speculums, and frames. Large photos leaned against the windows. One showed Annie dressed in vaudevillian lingerie, straddling a Harley, and singing into a Hitachi Magic Wand as if it were a microphone. Another showed Annie's partner, Beth, being stabbed in her nipple with a three-inch stiletto. I felt the pain in my own nipple. Maybe that was a sign that I was getting more in touch.

I felt awkward being there—she obviously had no time for me—but I was already there, so I couldn't back out. Beth entered carrying a huge flat-screen TV, followed by Annie waddling in with bags of food a minute later. Annie was older than I'd expected. I'd grown accustomed to looking at her Web site and her various items of photographic merchandise (not to mention the large photos now surrounding me), all of which were snapped years earlier. But age didn't seem to matter to her. She carried herself with pride and poise. She had a blue feather fluff ball in her short red hair. Black high heels matched her knee-length skirt. Did I mention her breasts? They're truly gigantic.

"Are you . . ." she said, looking at me.

SHE KNOWS A LOT ABOUT FEMALE ORGASM

"Mara," I said, not giving her a chance to get it wrong. "Yes."

"Right," she said. "Mara. Female orgasm, huh?"

The gallery owner, Tina, strolled inside just behind Annie. Tina had strawberry-blond hair and eyes like an animé character—all dewy and glistening against her powder-white skin. She wore an off-white sweater and was as flat-chested as Annie was stacked. She quietly rifled through papers on her desk.

Annie dropped her bags on top of a cluttered table. She asked if I could prepare the munchies. As I started unwrapping, Annie started pointing at the people around the room.

"She knows a lot about female orgasm," she said. "She knows a lot about female orgasm."

She went around the room, until the same phrase was said of everyone. "She knows A LOT about female orgasm." She was pointing to Tina this time. "Tina's in movies."

Annie had a lot to do before she was ready to make love to Duchamp the following day. She unpacked Hitachi Magic Wands, a boa, and an elaborate collage she had made out of her mammograms, which had revealed breast cancer just a few years ago. She was okay now.

"So you're in movies," I said to Tina.

"I'm a porn star," Tina said, putting her hands on her hips. Her screen name was Madison Young.

I knew what "being in movies" meant.

We started talking about her porn career. I hated that I was surprised she was a porn star, but I was. I admit it; I *was* surprised. Tina was originally from Ohio. She worked at Rainforest Café, or tried to work there, but didn't get the position, so she ended up with a job at the Lusty Lady, a unionized, worker-owned peep show co-op. From there things moved forward. Naked housekeeping. Masturbation shows. Then modeling for

Kink.com. Actual movies came next. Now she had her own Web sites. She said she liked it. I asked her how she funded her gallery.

"What you're asking," she said, "is how much anal sex for a feminist art space?"

"That works," I said.

She said it took ten anal scenes for the down payment and takes about three a month for the rent.

"Anal pays better," she said, "so I do both."

I needed to be busy for a little while. I dipped some carrots in hummus and had a section of an inside-out California roll. Tina looked over at Annie.

"Mine got broken," she told Annie. I hoped she wasn't talking about what I thought she was talking about.

"Oh," Annie said, empathetically, "they're too rough sometimes."

Annie caught my eye. "Those guys aren't like this," she said, putting her thumb and pointer finger together until the area between equaled the girth of a pencil. "No, this girl is amazing: she takes them like this," and she opened her fingers until a navel orange could fit through. "Big."

"Yeah, I need an anal vacation," Tina said. That was what she and "the girls" call it, she said, when they got sore.

"Do you have real orgasms when you shoot scenes?" I asked her.

"I demand it," she said. "Why fake it? Each orgasm is a revolutionary moment."

Maybe that was a stupid question because they rapidly dispatched me to Starbucks to fetch them lattes. Tina asked me if I wanted one; she was paying. I couldn't do it. I couldn't drink away her anal money. It wouldn't feel appropriate.

SHE KNOWS A LOT ABOUT FEMALE ORGASM

When I returned, Annie was yelling, "Where are my tit prints?"

No one answered her. She rummaged through folders and flipped through canvases. She finally found them. She'd dipped her tits in paint and then blotted them on matte paper. There were belly prints too, of her and Beth. "We're celebrating our new bodies," she said, patting her ample stomach.

I slid her tit prints into a binder and framed some sketches of her midsection. She thanked me for helping. Annie said she was sorry she didn't have time for an interview, so instead she gave me two of her DVDs for homework: *Amazing O* and *Sluts and Goddesses*.

Tina mentioned that she had to leave; the Porn Palace was having a Christmas party. The Porn Palace was the Kink.com headquarters, where Tina and her boyfriend worked; they shot a lot of bondage films there. She strutted toward the bathroom with a change of clothes—something gold and slinky.

"You should take Mara," Annie said.

Poor Tina. Even I felt bad for her as she made this awful face like kids make in elementary school when the teacher tells them they have to let the fat, acne-riddled kid join their dodgeball team.

"Mara should stay and help," said Tina. "You have so much to do here still."

"No," said Annie. "It's my fault I don't have time to interview. She should at least get to see something new."

"You need help, Annie," she said. "Look at this place."

"It's okay," Annie replied. "Take her."

"No, you need her," Tina said.

"No, take her."

"I think she should stay."

"She should go."

"She should stay."

"Go."

"Stay."

Everyone has their own agenda; I get it. But if I kept watching them, it would have been too sad, like seeing two kids with a ball playing keep-away from a gimp. Instead, I tried to seem indifferent, like two porn stars weren't trying to get rid of me. So I looked around more like I was following the pattern of an inebriated gnat smacking into windows.

Tina changed. She came out wearing a shimmery tank top and a black skirt that hugged her ass like mummy tape. Her hair was sleek. Her face was so smooth that she looked like a walking advertisement. I'm not sure exactly what she'd be advertising, but it didn't matter anyway—no matter what the product, a smooth face sells it. I'd been walking around the city in baggy jeans and faux Ugg boots for nine hours straight. I stunk, but I was going with her. She was reaching for the door, her hand lifting to say good-bye.

"Thanks for the invite," I said, following behind her.

Tina and I stood outside the Porn Palace. I wasn't on the list, so she had to call her porn-star boyfriend, James, outside. He and the bouncer questioned what I was writing my book on. I'd never wanted to be writing a book about something else—*anything* else— as much as I did right then.

I confessed: no orgasm.

The Porn Palace had many film sets: a dungeon, a chain room, a jail cell, a half-moon-shaped water bondage tank, a small farmhouse. My favorite was "the wall of inspiration," which was a wall of toys—everything from whips to gas masks. Sir B in Jersey City wouldn't have needed the enema kit if he saw this; he would have shat his pants at the bounty present. They had everything. James told me they made two million dollars a month on their movies.

SHE KNOWS A LOT ABOUT FEMALE ORGASM

There are a lot of kinky folk out there.

Tina introduced me to another porn star, Adrienne. She had dark eyebrows but really blond hair. She had on pedal pusher pants and a red French manicure. She stood with a guy who ran, and was the star of, the Web site Hogtied.com, which specialized in movies featuring women tied up.

"I give women orgasms for a living," he said in a gruff voice. "Best job ever!"

Tina said she's had some of her best with him. Her boyfriend walked by and spanked her butt right then; her cheeks were so oblivious to gravity that they seemed to reach out and slap him back.

Tina said that I should stay there for a week, and if I did, I would certainly have an orgasm. The Hogtied guy said they'd give me an orgasm in nice ways.

"I like it with a Magic Wand, a fist, and some rope," said Tina.

"So if you did it to me," I asked, "would those things be used?"

"Those are nice," he said.

"Nice," I said, repeating him. Maybe he'd think I was an echo and leave me alone.

We posed with a Real Doll, one of the life-size silicone dolls a person can have sex with. In the spirit of the holidays, it was dressed up like Mrs. Claus, but with a beer bottle shoved up the vaginal canal. A guy snapped a Polaroid of us and tucked it in a cardboard frame.

We all gathered in the dungeon. They were giving out awards for best editing and showing trailers of movies on the screen. Tina was to the right of me; her boyfriend behind her. As the presentation began, he rubbed her nipples until they stood up like two little teepees under her shirt. There was a brief clip of her; she was being trained to be a submissive. At that moment, when I saw a toilet-bowl perspective of her—yes, the camera seemed to be in the toilet—naked and vomiting, I was sure I'd made the right decision in not going back to Sir B.

I walked around but soon returned to Tina and Adrienne. They were in a corner drinking vodka and cranberry juice. They were talking about how Tina had lost her clit ring down some guy named Mark's throat during a shoot. Then they got back to the finer points of anal; they thought it somehow hit their G-spot best. Adrienne, as it happens, had actually visited Dr. Matlock, the Box Cutter, when she got her vagina ripped on a really big dick.

"Small world," I said.

The way she looked at me said, *You had your vagina ripped by a big dick too?*

"Oh, I know who Dr. Matlock is," I said. "I mean, I've met him before."

She continued. She said the surgery didn't work. She still hurt and preferred it up the ass. The big-schlonged dude didn't even say he was sorry. But she still had a clit and an asshole, so she said she was happy.

I was beginning to feel like a stalker. I was keeping so close to them that if I had a penis, it'd probably be up them both. They'd file for a restraining order. I wouldn't be able to go within five feet of them. I didn't like that feeling, of needing, of impinging. But look at me, I had stalked them right into a corner. They were behind a pillar, shadowed by some large speakers. Had they been trying to hide from me? Must be bad mojo to have a nonclimaxer at your pornography headquarters. I felt like the anti-pornography. I tell you, I kicked myself out—after a slice of decadent chocolate cake and a couple vodka cranberry juices. I kicked myself out. I just couldn't do it to them anymore.

I went to bed. A streetlamp shone through the blinds, orangeish on my sheets. And then I saw the blink blink blink in the corner.

SHE KNOWS A LOT ABOUT FEMALE ORGASM

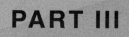

PART III

FLUMMOXED

By the time I awoke the following morning, my aunt had already left the apartment. I stepped, alone, onto her porch with a mug of coffee. The bay was murky with fog just like my coffee was with milk, just like I was with a deviated thinking process. It seemed my mind, somehow, had stopped thinking straight; I had two simultaneous internal monologues running and I'd stayed on the sidelines, watching them duke it out. Something had happened, but I wasn't sure what it was yet. This caused my subsequent interviews to be somewhat muddled.

It wasn't until two days later, when I was talking to Fiona, that I made sense of things. I was scrolling Web pages while she talked, but then I stopped and stared at the rug. I followed the spiral patterns with my eyes. It clicked. When she said, "Shit," it clicked. She said, "Shit, it's not what I thought."

But first, let me catch up on the day before. I had watched my baby cousin for a few hours. She wanted to play Superman. She jumped from the sofa, and as I caught her, I thought, If it had in fact happened—if the right wires had been tripped—wouldn't I now be yearning for my own jumping sack of joy? But I wasn't yearning. Not at all. Actually, I was just hoping that *this* sack of joy wouldn't poop before her parents came home.

So, maybe what I'd felt was *a* sensation but not *the* sensation. Yeah, it couldn't have been it. It wasn't. If it *had* happened, I'd be grounded, on track. I'd now have a desire to settle down and possibly even subscribe to a magazine like *Consumer Reports* or maybe even *Sunset*. Besides, what had actually occurred couldn't even be called volcanic, let alone eruptive. But then again, it *was* something fluttery and rather unique.

Soon I was at the Oakland Bart station to meet for an interview. A black Jetta hugged the curb. A cigarette hung from the driver's fingertips as she blew smoke out the window. She had a short pixie haircut, auburn. She wore a green furry hat. She was lanky, and when she pulled up her sunglasses, I could tell she'd had a late night. She carried baggage around her eyes like The Collector does on my Brooklyn porch. I guess we all store our baggage somewhere; mine was thwacking around in my brain at the moment. Thwacks were my inner ambiance.

It was Dorrie Lane. I didn't expect the inventor of pastel puppet twats to look so edgy. My expectations were leading me astray these days anyway. I stepped inside and belted up. I couldn't remember anymore why we'd gotten together, but I knew I had badgered her to get there. She pulled into the street. "Oh, goddess!" she said, as a car sped past. She said goddess instead of god.

She drove toward a popular little lesbian brunch spot near Berkeley. Trance music was playing softly. As I tapped my foot, I noticed I was off-beat. And I looked uneasy; I know I did because I saw my face in the side-view mirror. My nostrils were disobediently flared, and the way I was furrowing constructed a Frida Kahlo unibrow.

When given no direction from her interviewer, Dorrie, the interviewee, got on her soapbox. This is what one woman said when she had a soapbox: Why can't we honor women as the true creators? Why aren't young girls taught that in school? If we respected the vulva, there wouldn't be rape. It's a transgression against women, which is the very place we all come from.

"Oh, my goddess," Dorrie said, looking at the menu. "I'm starved." I drank coffee. She ate. She flirted with our tattooed waitress while the only question that came to my mind—How do you know when you've had an orgasm?—just seemed too gauche to utter, especially when speaking to a woman with a silver vulva ring on her finger. It's unfair. Guys have that very convenient indicator when they've had an orgasm: the corresponding jism. But women's seem to work on an abstract continuum.

On the way to her place, I stared at that vulva ring, the one I had seen months ago on her Web site and sworn I would never wear. I actually thought it was pretty classy now. The vulva, that little fucker, was really growing on me. They do that, vulvas; they grow on people, especially Dorrie.

She lived in a converted warehouse. There was pussy everywhere: vulva mouse pad, vulva jewelry, colorful vulva puppets overflowing in baskets. There was a new model minivulva she demonstrated for me. She told me about Eve Ensler, the creator of *The Vagina Monologues*, and explained that her show is named wrong. The vagina is the canal. "It connotes sexual intercourse with a penis," Dorrie said, "the heterosexual vanilla way."

"Clit Conversations!" she said. "That's what it should be called."

Dorrie puffed on her cigarette and exhaled the room all smoky. I took a cigarette instead of one of the cookies she'd laid out. You'd think that I had forgotten I feared death, the way I was inhaling.

You'd think I had forgotten myself. As I sifted through the cunt jewelry, my brain floated luxuriously in its own fluid, lounging on a nicotine rush. I bought two vulva rings, one for me and one for Fiona. I put mine on my left-hand ring finger.

Dorrie took me back to the train. Things kept feeling weird; they weren't feeling normal. I was running late for Annie's energy orgasm séance. I wasn't in the mood to make energy love to a dead man at the moment, but I went anyway because I never let me not wanting to do something get in the way of me not enjoying it, especially if it was marked on my agenda. Plus, I wanted to learn more. I just didn't know what that more was yet.

But the next day, it clicked—all these contradictory feelings clicked—when Fiona called and said, "Shit, it's not what I thought," and I followed the rug's patterns around with my orbs.

But before I get to that, let me catch up on the séance. They'd transformed the gallery overnight. The photos were hung, the tit prints neatly stacked. I bounced around to the different installations. I spotted Tina. I stayed away; I didn't want to stalk. In tribute to Duchamp's readymade artwork—like the urinal he turned upside down, named *Fountain*, and then signed R. Mutt—Annie displayed a Hitachi and signed it R. Muff. A framed picture of Duchamp hung below a bronzed pair of panties, which once belonged to Rose Selavy, a pseudonym he used for himself when dressed as a woman. The centerpiece of the show was a film showing on the flat-screen television. It was called *Big Nudes Descending a Stairway* and was inspired by Duchamp's *Nude Descending a Staircase*. It showed a naked Annie and Beth, big bellies and all, walking slowly down spiraling Parisian steps. It was on repeat mode. The only sounds were from the thuds of their soles.

By eight p.m., the tiny space was crammed with people. Annie quieted the masses; the séance was set to begin. Everyone circled around a massage table set up in the center of the room. It was covered with a heavy oriental rug on which a large man named Ted lay down. He was the medium. A young woman, dressed in vintage garb, began singing operatically to channel Duchamp's spirit into him.

"Marceeeeeeeel," she sang. "Maaaaaaaaarcelllllll Duuuuuuuchaaaaaaaaamp."

We all held hands as a cat hopped in between the medium's legs. It sat with its butt against his crotch and swatted, with its orange-striped tail, at his genitals. Laughter erupted; everyone figured Duchamp must have been in the body by then.

Annie began breathing heavily, and everyone else followed suit. They screeched and hollered. I didn't do anything. The room got steamy and the windows fogged. I watched the steam turn into droplets and trickle down the glass. Clamminess exuded from the hand holding mine. People fanned their faces as their cheeks went flush.

Then it was done. Annie declared it over. We'd made love to Marcel Duchamp.

That was the easiest lovemaking I'd ever done. I should get people to do it for me more often.

As Annie's guests started leaving, she was finally ready to help me. She was sweet. She wanted to counsel Mia or Mara or Mia or Mara, whichever young woman it was who needed an orgasm.

I followed her to the massage table. She pulled herself up and started making grunting noises, breathing hard and flailing her arms in circles to the side of her head like she was winding up her own pair of Princess Leia's pigtails.

Then Annie told me to hop up; it was my turn to try the fire-breath energy orgasm. If partnered with sex, she said, the breathing technique would leave me satisfied every time. I climbed onto the table. I felt like the bull's-eye for everyone's stares. I got uncomfortable—self-conscious—and wanted to hop down.

The feeling reminded me of how I'd always felt when I'd tried to share my sexuality with another person. I'd be in bed with a guy, he'd be turning me on, flipping my switches and fingering my insides, and I'd start to feel something, like a quivering in my thighs and lower spine that could potentially lead to previously unknown heights of sensation, so I'd hold on tighter, or I'd inch away so that he couldn't continue—so that I wouldn't lose control and he wouldn't have control over me. And if I lost it, I feared my body would go spastic. Feminine grace, I imagined, could not be maintained while the involuntary musculature reigned. I worried more about what he would see than what I would feel.

And now all these people in the gallery were looking at me up on that table. I was supposed to be loose with Annie guiding me in my grunting and supposed to be just fine losing my faculties in front of everyone. I would have looked unattractive in my unraveling, in my intimate unveiling.

But the other night, after the Porn Palace party, I had been alone. I didn't care what I looked like. I just wanted to feel something real. I wanted to show myself that I could be a completely independent girl. I didn't need to depend on someone else to turn me on. That's when I saw the blink blink blinking in the corner.

I never could share myself very well, I suppose. And I still couldn't, apparently. Because I finally had this tremendously orgasmic woman's undivided attention, putting forth her energy to help me reach my climax, and all I wanted to do was depart. I hopped down, off the massage table.

"Everyone has orgasms when they're little kids," Annie said, as I went for the exit. "Your problem is you're trying to control it."

I left.

So it was the following day when I was at my computer that Fiona called. She was in Wisconsin. I was in my cousin's apartment, practicing my methods of procrastination. Eric, my sacred whore, had just IM-ed me and then immediately signed off.

Eric: appear/tickle/pounce/poof!

What the hell did that mean? Fiona brimmed with excitement. She could barely stop her rush of words for the necessary inhale. She started reciting passages from *The Fountainhead*. I got up and paced the house. She'd got all wrapped up in capitalistic diatribes and topped herself off with a smattering of *Eat, Pray, Love* self-finding manifesto. She was finding herself in paragraphs. She was pointing out sentences that resonated most.

"Fi," I said, "what are you trying to say exactly?"

She said she had had an epiphany. "Shit," she said, "it's all just not what I thought."

I was silent for a second.

"You there?" she asked.

And that's when I kind of realized I'd just gone through a good two full days of orgasm denial. One of my two running monologues had been saying that I'd had the orgasm, while the other said to ignore that crotch indigestion I'd felt and go out and interview, business as usual, until I found the orgasm I was *supposed* to have—the one that I'd heard would feel like fireworks were detonating in my crotch.

"I don't think it's what I thought, either," I said to Fiona.

Then I went on to elaborate what had happened with me and my purple vibrator, which was actually green. I told her that that night, when I got back from the Porn Palace party, I'd seen the blink blink blinking in the corner. I already felt ridiculous for not doing what it seemed like the whole world, at least the world I'd found myself in, seemed to revolve around doing. I had finally become desensitized; orgasms were the norm. I wouldn't let pornography reject me so easily. So I unplugged the vibe and wouldn't give up. A Luddite at heart, I got my paw down there like Betty had counseled. I poked and prodded and stroked and squeezed and rubbed and squinted and held my breath until . . . until . . . well . . . until my crotch kind of sneezed. My biggest indicator that this was the thing I'd been looking for, even though it was nothing like what I expected, was that I felt tiny contractions—miniature unintentional Kegels—in tandem with a warm, fluttery commotion near Clitty Rose's canal region.

"Congratulations!" Fiona said. She was truly pleased.

"But that's it?" I asked. "That's an orgasm?"

She told me the sensation, for her, is different each time. Sometimes her orgasms just feel like warm wax pouring slowly throughout her insides while other times her body reacts as if she'd stuck her finger in a live socket. She said it's not possible to have the same orgasm twice. Her explanation reminded me of how she talks about each new lover: I've never felt this way before, she always says. Maybe each orgasm, on its own, is a tiny love affair.

But I couldn't help feeling like my orgasm must have been clogged. It needed some Metamucil-type equivalent to help it move along. Not only was the sensation underwhelming, but I'd also expected more to happen as a result of its attainment. I'd planned to be enlightened, damn it. When I went out onto my aunt's porch the morning following my first successful masturbation, I'd anticipated a whole new clarity, but even my coffee had been murky. I had closed my eyes. The passing cloud patches fickly shielded the sun, constantly changing the hues of red I saw under my eyelids, making me aware of both inside and outside simultaneously. I had even more questions than when I had started this journey. Maybe just having an orgasm—becoming orgasmic—wasn't enough.

When I got off the phone, I knew that what I'd previously expected to be the finish line turned out to be only step one.

I KNOW WE'RE IN THE MIDDLE, BUT THIS IS REALLY JUST THE BEGINNING

So Satya, the *dakini*. I didn't really know what I was getting into. I had read her Web page and all, but I still had no idea what she would try on me. All I knew for sure was that her name, in Sanskrit, meant truth. So I showed up at her temple at five p.m. I was leaving the following evening. She wasn't quite ready for me, so I waited, sitting on the curb, getting ready to be traumatized. I watched the sunset slide down a three-story building. I kept thinking, "I never thought I'd be waiting by someone's door to pay for sexual contact." But I was learning things weren't always what I thought. She let me in. She wore a silk robe and gave me a hot cup of tea. And then we sat down for a while. We talked. I couldn't really look her in the eye. I giggled at the wrong moments. I picked that little bump by my hairline. When I get nervous, I just keep picking at it more. Disgusting. I've irritated it and its retribution has been to slightly expand its dimensions. So I picked as we talked and I sipped my tea. I felt weird being there. What *should* I be acting like? There never was a sitcom that taught me how to act at a Tantra session. It was dim. There were candles lit. Trance music played softly. Satya asked me questions and was intrigued with my quest. I told her that I had already had my first orgasm. "You don't water a plant only once," she said. One of her teachers, Margo Anand, said that there are as many different orgasms as there are stars in the sky, so I had no less exploration ahead of me; this was really just the beginning. I agreed. She said she had gone through the same kind of journey, long ago. She was now thirty-two.

Her temple was white-walled. A couple of paintings. Some oriental rugs and a massage table wrapped with towels. Screens partitioned the table from the rest of the room. There was a little altar and a sofa low to the floor. Cushions, lots of cushions. She was voluptuous in her silk robe. Her hair fell in long brown ringlets, and she had eyes that focused really well—totally clear. She told me that most people try to separate all that is below the waist from what is above. Tantra is the practice that opens up a portal between and unites them both.

Then she asked if I wanted to be naked. What was normal, I asked? She said people were naked sometimes, but I could do whatever I wanted. "There is no normal," she said. I wished she would just say what normal was so I could do it.

It was time to begin. She asked me to leave my contribution in the vessel by the candle and to make a wish. I left the going rate, three hundred dollars (that sounds like a lot, but men pay twice that). I put the money in the pot and lingered there, trying to find just the right wish, because if I was paying that much, I'd better get all that I could out of it, even if it was abstract. My wish couldn't be put into words; it was more of a sense.

We stood face to face and breathed. She asked if I wanted a hug. Normal? Okay. Sure. It was a good hug. We did some yoga moves. I bent down and touched my toes. Then I squatted. I was supposed to be feeling my breath. I always have trouble with that. She asked if I was gay or bisexual. I said no. Then I felt like I had to qualify why I was seeing a woman if I wasn't gay. "Because I was referred and thought it would be more comfortable." And, in fact, it was. I think—well, despite the not-being-able-to-look-into-her-retinas deal. Then we both breathed. My hand was on her chest and hers on mine. She asked if I was going to get naked and I said maybe. Normal?

She left the room and I decided that, for three hundred dollars, I should make her see the parts of my body I was frightened to. I was paying enough to have someone endure my butt pimple. So I stripped and lay facedown. She started rubbing my back with oil. Her roommate on the floor above was doing laundry and I could hear the shit tumbling around in the dryer. She told me to breathe. She said that I should make noises to release whatever it was I was feeling. I suck rather horribly at noises. She was proud I never used them to fake orgasms though. She said fake orgasms just got you further from your goal. Rori says goals aren't everything; that's what I was thinking. Then I was thinking that I liked how she rubbed me. Then she took everything off. "I like to do this natural," she said. And natural meant nothing but a g-string and her back tattoo. Oh, hoop earrings too. It felt nice for her breasts to cup my head. Her hair tickled my back. My butt was in the air, totally out there. She started touching my vulva in sweeps every once in a while. And it was really nice. It was just like another body part, a nook to massage. It was like finding that nook in between your shoulder blades that never gets touched and it suddenly gets stroked and it wakes up a little bit.

She told me to visualize the Fountain of Amrita, which is a fancy name for female ejaculate, and I gave her a frightened stare over my shoulder. She said I could visualize other things, too, so

I did. I thought up a nice, overly chlorinated (you know, like the smell practically singes your nostrils) fountain washing over me. And then she flipped me over. My beaver winked at her. I was worried about being turned on. I mean, it made sense because she'd been stroking it, but then again, she's a girl and I was straight, and what if that confused me? She continued massaging and said I could touch her. I didn't. I stayed very still. She had amazing breasts. Some of the most amazing I've seen, and I wanted to touch them . . . but was that normal? What is normal? I can't function without societal expectations.

After more stimulation of my clit, she asked if I wanted a G-spot massage. This was desensitization at its finest; my dad would have been so proud of me. So I said I had to go pee first, and when I got off the table I felt like my head was a helium balloon that was floating away. My eardrums started to crackle (I'd been laying off the Q-tips, too, so I didn't think that was the problem). When I got back to her, I felt an echo in my head, and she sounded like there was a funnel in between her mouth and my ears with parrots flying around in the chasm. When I closed my eyes, I saw stars. I started to count them to know how many more orgasms I'd have. And then I lay back down and she sprayed a ton of oil on me and I tried to express my feeling about that with a noise on my next exhalation. Eeehh ehhhh aahhhaa. It came out like the wheeze of a deflating tire. And she rubbed in the oil and touched my third eye. She had great touch. It went deep. She knew what she was doing. And so she tried to stick her finger in, but I was so anxious that when she placed it at the introitus I clenched. My fists were tight and I bet my anus was about the size of a goldfish's . . . And she tried to get in and I tried to relax and it was a rough moment complete with squinty eyes and furrowed brow. She got one finger in. I asked her if she could feel my G-spot yet and she said not quite yet. She needed two fingers. She tried to put the other one in but it wouldn't fit. I felt like such a fucking novice. I thought about my new porn star acquaintances, who would be embarrassed for me. They were all about fisting. So she had her one finger up there and she was looking at my vulva and I realized that she was probably the only person besides me, Noam, and my gyno to see Miss Clitty Rose so up close. I felt like I was opening up; I was finally letting someone in. Maybe I could share me after all. And I wondered why that body part was any different from any other. It should have been even more out in the open, maybe, because it gave so much pleasure. I mean, really, why is the part of the body that probably needs the most release and can, in fact, give the body the most pleasure the one part that is bound by so many laws? And then she started rubbing my G-spot. Or what she said was my G-spot. I'm still skeptical because my aunt said G-spots are mumbo-jumbo. A lot of people still think that. And I felt like I had to pee again. For me, the G-spot rub canceled out the good feelings of the clit. Zola said the G-spot released traumas and memories, so I was waiting to break down and cry or have a shooting gush of amrita or some crazy epiphany. But I didn't. Instead my lips—my actual lips, the ones on my mouth—got all stuck and I couldn't breathe through my mouth anymore. My upper lip curled and twitched. Then I felt pressure on my left rib cage. Everything felt tingly, but not the same kind of tingly as when a body part has been asleep, a different kind. I was more conscious of my insides than ever. Her fingers, at that moment, somehow felt like they were part of me. The sensation, though not orgasmic, was more intricate and foreign than my first climax had been. Then I thought I was hyperventilating again. I had fucked up my body by breathing too much. I was used to breathing just enough to get by. And so I stopped breathing really deep and all that feeling didn't go away. And she was really jamming down there, but the other finger still wouldn't go in. She said to stay with the feeling and soon new neural passages would be built to sustain it. I'd soon be orgasming easier and stronger—no genital indigestion but a full-on four-diamond crotchular express ride. This was just the beginning, she said. She gave me hope. And then she pulled out her finger and she came close to me. Her head floated above mine, her hair pulled back in a ponytail and just her hoops hanging down. Her breasts were practically resting on my chest. And it was nice, and intimate, but not gross. I kind of wished that I knew what she knew and that I could just treat my friends to a lovely night like this, but it's not like that. Most of them would freak out. So would I. She asked me to explain my sensations to her. I did and she said she wasn't surprised. She said I would, if I worked hard enough, begin to harness my sexual energy—my kundalini. She said right now it was so strong because it was like a volcano that hadn't erupted. I didn't let it go anywhere but inside. I didn't make noises and I didn't move around. She said a lot of people looked like they were swimming on the table when she did what she had just done. Now she tells me what normal is, after it's all over.

I'd wondered, while I had all the sensations, if sex was like a drug. I'd never been very good with drugs. I had always felt things too much and I wondered if maybe I felt sex too much. Maybe that's why I had shut down. I feared getting consumed by visceral reactions and losing myself to my bottom half. I didn't want to get lost. Satya, though, made it seem like getting lost might be part of being found.

She walked around the table, stroking me softly for the cool-down. She said I was like a rosebud. She could feel my energy starting to flow. "You're definitely on a journey," she said. Even though I knew I was on a journey, it felt good to be validated. Validations are always good. And then she hovered over me, her face lit by the candle flames. She smiled and her eyes twinkled and her makeup shimmered. She said she was proud of me; I was brave for my first time. I knew I'd progressed. Though I didn't have an orgasm during the session, something maybe even more extraordinary occurred. She'd stirred up a hunger, an energy, maybe it could be called a desire, the essence of which, for a long time, had settled beneath my awareness. Then she wrapped me up in a blanket. I wasn't traumatized.

KNOCKOFFS

I was on the overnight Greyhound bus heading north for my stay with the Orgasm People. I was off to Orgasm Camp.

They had originally moved to the middle of nowhere, in part to enjoy their orgasmic-community-living way of life without society there to judge and misinterpret it. So to preserve their privacy, I agreed to change not only their names but their location. We'll call it Pussy Willow Ranch.

I'd walked up and down the bus a number of times, trying to find a seat. I felt much more normal than I had in a long time, just by observing my surrounding bus mates. Greyhound was notorious for attracting misfits. One woman glowered at me as I watched her eat white stuff out of a stuffed latex glove. Seriously.

"Are you a hippie?" asked a bedraggled boy eating Doritos; cheese particles were stuck to his pencil-thin mustache.

"No," I said.

"Oh, I was going to let you sit with me," he said. "Never mind."

Not being a hippie had never thrilled me more.

I sat by the first person who didn't say anything to me, a man passed out with a roll of knockoff Fig Newtons on his lap. The bus was soon under way.

My last day in San Francisco, I'd met up with Tallulah Sulis. She owns the video production company Juicy Mama Productions and was the director of the slightly nauseating female ejaculation film *Divine Nectar*, which Zola had assigned me to watch in New York. Tallulah's clit lore about Betty was amusing—she said she had heard Betty's clit was as big as a pinkie finger—but it was Tallulah's preoccupation with gushes via la vulva (she even said her name, in the American Choctaw language, means "leaping water") that actually got to me. I actually kind of cared about female ejaculation after talking to her.

"Women have been told ejaculation is something they're not capable of," she'd said. "They are made to feel ashamed and embarrassed of it, but this is an absolute scientific fact: women *do* ejaculate! They are healed through the reclamation of their gushiness!"

Every woman has the anatomy to ejaculate, she said. Any wet spot during sex or orgasm could be evidence of a squirt; it doesn't always go projectile-style, she said. Female ejaculation isn't a skill exactly, but some just master the technique and can propel their streams to greater lengths. To hone your ability to gush, she said, takes practice and complete surrender in a highly aroused state. "Also time spent massaging the G-spot," she added. "You have to kind of mill it."

"For me, it went from a tiny, tiny bit," she continued, "to me being able to release huge amounts. Then I began gushing like fountains and rivers and I'd wet entire beds and it'd just be airborne; it'd be everywhere. But remember, it's not about the amount, it's about the release. I think of it as giving birth to orgasm."

If I had been in a more sentimental mindset, I might have even teared up—well, after I made her explain how female ejaculation isn't urine. She said there've been studies and that she'd also performed her own test: "It doesn't taste like pee at all," she said.

I was convinced.

When she left she told me, all excited, that the new Erotic Revolution was occurring. The feminine waters, she said, would usher it in. I wished her good luck with that.

The bus got quiet and I suddenly felt sleepy. I pulled off my shoes and crossed my feet on the seat. I rubbed them. With my finger, I outlined the scars from my bunion surgery. I remembered Fred licking them. And I wondered why sex was any different than a lick, than patting someone's shoulder or running barefoot on the earth. Wasn't it all just vibration, friction—membrane to membrane, molecules to molecules—in some sense? I guess it was something Tallulah had said that had me pondering. "The more you can expand the meaning of orgasm," she'd said, "the more you can be liberated by orgasm."

When I was on Satya's table, I strained to figure out what normal was; I wanted to be normal so badly that I subverted my authenticity. But I'd never truly been genuine during sex. I was too busy trying to figure out what was "right"—the right noises, moves, reactions, and emotions. In the past I'd had the desire to yell, to chant, to sleep, to weep, but instead I tried to figure out what "sexy" looked like. I had detached myself from the act so that I could have unencumbered sex like "liberated" girls. The opposite occurred: I became locked inside myself. I became the opposite of gushiness.

I'd felt almost guiltier for keeping my orgasm from Rori than I did about keeping it from myself. When I finally divulged the disappointing climax to her over the phone, she didn't register it as a bad thing. She told me to apply my crotch sneeze to how I lived in the world. If I could listen to what pleased my body, even slightly, then I could start to listen more deeply to my desires. I could tell who turned me on and trust my senses. I'd know what I wanted and what I didn't want without filtering it through my very picky gray matter. In other words, I wouldn't have to depend on nutritional information to figure out which flavor cookie I wanted.

My seat buddy continued to sleep. His snore kept coming closer to my ear, and his head hovered just above my shoulder. I'm afraid of stranger slobber, so I moved my shoulder down and his head dropped, bobbed up, dropped down, and then convulsed to the other side where it could rest.

I nodded off to sleep.

I awoke as the sun crept above the peak of Mount Shasta. The rustle of my neighbor's cookie package woke me; they'd been on his lap the whole trip. I was hungry—I wanted one of *those* cookies—so I started a conversation. Santos was a thirty-two-year-old Guatemalan man. He only spoke Spanish. He told me he was going to drive a car all the way from Portland to Guatemala for his congregation. It wasn't long before the conversation turned to spousal hunting. He told me to find a husband immediately and then explained how missionaries had told him all about the Apocalypse. I told him I didn't do Bible stuff and was even more unsure about husband stuff. He said it wasn't too late. He offered me a knockoff Fig Newton from his stores as consolation for the eternity I'd be burning in hell. I happily broke the knockoff into bits and swallowed it down.

I could still repent, he said. God would still accept me. I nodded as crumbs speckled my lap. Santos looked at me in disbelief. To him, I fit in perfectly on that bus; I was one of those crazy Greyhound misfits. Who wouldn't be considered crazy for eschewing sound advice and choosing a different path?

We have more choices than we choose to accept.

ORGASM CAMP

Pussy Willow Ranch, December 9, 10 p.m. PWCT

I'm supposed to be masturbating right now. Masturbation is my homework assignment for tonight, but I haven't gotten to it yet. I'm going to do it. I can't report to the teachers tomorrow that the dog ate my homework. The dog can't eat this kind of homework.

I'm sitting in bed at the camper's cottage, about a three-minute walk from the brown house where I'd just eaten dinner with all the Orgasm People, or the OP for short. That's where they all sleep.

I have to DO myself right now. That's what they call their method of orgasm: Deliberate Orgasm, DO for short, which seems to have metamorphosed into its own verb. You can DO, be DONE, or presently be DOing. DO involves clit stroking, much like One-Taste's OM. More or less, they use a honed finger-strum to take a woman on an orgasmic ride—peaks and valleys, twists, turns, loops. Any pattern she's swinging seems to be a go as long as the finger is smack-dab clitorally located.

The Orgasm People live for the DO. For the twelve of them—three men and nine women—the DO is what they do. They don't have jobs. It seems they even make their money from DOing; they DO on DVDs and sell them as sex education videos. It's all female orgasm all the time, and if they have extra time, they work on remodeling their kitchen and eat fantastic food. Doesn't sound bad, right?

But something's strange. It's like they've spent so much time by themselves in the woods researching their bodies that they somehow even know mine better than I do. As we sat down to shallow bowls of beef stew, just a little while ago, I felt see-through. They intuit everything. They even claim to feel one another's orgasms—so in touch with their own sensation that they feel the runoff from others' too.

The laws of nature, as I've come to know them, aren't working here. The Orgasm People even changed their time zone. They call it PWCT—Pussy Willow Creek Time—after the small body of water that snakes through their property. They live an hour ahead of the rest of California so they get more daylight, and because the nearest civilization is an hour away, they can leave for errands at the time they want to arrive. Their time isn't the only thing they have changed; they also refuse to believe that female orgasm is what about 99.99 percent of the population believes it entails. But I'll get to that in a second.

Now I'm back to the beef stew dinner, and the truth is, I'm paranoid. I feel they could burrow their eyes into my being and know what I'm thinking. Getting sex stuff squared away has made their communication channels clearer or something.

They know that when they ask how I slept I'm wondering if they are going to DO me. When they ask me how the food is, I'm like, wow, how did they get such amazing breasts? The way the women frame their cleavage with clothing makes their breasts seem not like mere body parts but valuable accessories that bedeck their chests like diamond-packed jewelry. When they ask if I want coffee, I'm thinking, How many orgasms did she have today, and if I had that many, would my saunter be as smooth, my air so graceful, my being so centered, and my metabolism so fast?

"Yes, with sugar and milk," I answer.

When they ask me if I want to go on a walk, I wonder what they've all been through. Where do they sleep? Whom do they sleep with? What is a romantic relationship to them? There are no wedding pictures on the mantel; in fact, I don't even think they have a mantel. Where's their mantel?

"Yes, a walk sounds nice."

They know what I'm thinking and then they will go over it later, as a group. *Do you know what Mara was thinking? She was really crazy last night at dinner. When she was peeling that orange, she was thinking, "I want Collin to DO me."* They say that when a man wants to have sex with a woman, the only way he will have that idea is if the woman sees it as a possibility; otherwise that idea wouldn't pop into his head. Women are the ones with the turn-on; men just react to it. So then I'm thinking they must all be thinking that I would have sex with them or be DONE by them. I hope they aren't thinking that because it wouldn't be true, and then I start to realize that it *is* true. I'm thinking about DOing all the time. Then I try to make the thought go away. Go away. I think about the preserves. Those yummy apricot preserves. Yes, focus. Focus. Will they DO me? No, stop. Preserves. Radicchio. Asparagus spears.

Then I can't stop thinking about the food because it has never tasted so delicious—the food is fuckable. They raise their own livestock and grow their own produce on their swath of forest, so in the middle of nowhere that there's nothing but trees to see. I've never consciously tried to penetrate a baguette, steamy and doughy, in quite the manner I attempted at their table tonight. It was like each bite I'd taken before that point was a bastardized version of true flavor, and now the bulbous nerve endings protruding from my tongue made love to the food in its honest form. I guess a part of my taking up coitus with the cuisine was also because I was feeling left out. I wanted to make love to *something*.

You should see them, these Orgasm People. They are always laughing, though I never get the jokes. I think they've all suffered some kind of orgasm overdose. It's hard to trust people who are so happy; it feels like they must have screws loose. I picked at my little forehead bump. Thinking. That little bump was so comforting; I could depend on it being there. I watched all their cheeks flushing.

Oh, they don't wear makeup, either. Artificial pigment is turn-on forgery, and they want to know the truth about how turned on each of us is at each moment. I wear makeup at ACE Bar; all the cocktail waitresses do. We make our money by camouflaging our turn-off. Many women do.

There are two older men, in their sixties, in the rooms next door to me. They are my orgasm co-campers, and they are supposed to be masturbating right now, too. I can hear one of them wanking away. Honestly, I'm happy he's getting rowdy with himself, but I think I'd rather have one of the Orgasm People's billy goats in bed with me, baaaa-ing into my ear, than have to listen to this guy's moaning. The sound of other people's pleasure, especially that of strangers or new acquaintances, is oddly discomfiting. I feel like I'm not supposed to be here.

I have a glob of lube and some dew towels in front of me (they call washcloths dew towels). Dolly, in her French maid uniform, gave me the masturbation accoutrements after dinner. Yesterday, when I first saw her in her uniform before class, I could only ogle. Up to that point, all the Orgasm ladies—aged thirty to their mid-fifties—looked like soccer moms. They'd be the ones taking casseroles out of the oven for a potluck.

But Dolly: the black ruffled skirt reached just below her bum, and fishnet stockings covered her legs the rest of the way down to her leather heels. Her bust popped out from her low neckline like batter rising over the rim of a cupcake tin. I waited until the teachers entered the room and then asked why Dolly was dressed like a Halloween version of a French maid. Neil, who seemed to be the silverback of the pack, looked at me like I was an idiot.

"It's fun, isn't it?" he said. He pulled out a pocketknife. It opened with a *thwack*. The blade looked sharp enough to make sashimi out of me.

"Yeah," I said, shooting him a placating smile. "Fun."

I found out that fun, in their world, is the number one reason for doing something, anything, everything. That made way more sense than I was ready to admit at that moment. I'm used to doing things because I have to, because I'm supposed to.

Neil fell backward into a big sofa chair, and with the knife he began contentedly shoveling out the underside of his nails. Neil and three women—the instructors—sat across from me and my co-campers, petting home-cured goat pelts placed in swatches against the sofa's armrests, as they delivered the lesson by reading line after line out of a three-ringed binder. Class was dry. No genitals. All clothes. Only words. Lots of words. Over the course of the weekend, I sat through sixteen hours' worth of words. The whole while, there were undertones of submissive role-play as Dolly served them tea on hand and knee.

ORGASM CAMP

"Everyone is sexually lame," Neil had started. "And everyone thinks they have issues fucking."

I sure was glad he had gotten that out of the way.

Neil had a stock of amazing sound-bites. Here's another: "A guy not willing to take a used tampon out of a woman's pussy with his teeth doesn't deserve to get his cock sucked."

It was oddly empowering, even though I would never let a dude do that.

But back to masturbation. I should really get going. It's getting late and my next-door neighbor is starting to quiet down. It's my turn, and all of a sudden it's not that hard anymore, because do you know what these Orgasm People do? Even though they are professional comers and can come for an hour—which I'll be seeing tomorrow during the OIC (Observation of Intense Coming)—they've changed the definition of orgasm so that any woman who has a crotch can have an orgasm any time she wants. They say an orgasm occurs the moment the genitals feel better than the rest of the body.

In the seventies, Masters and Johnson declared that female orgasm is marked by three to fifteen uterine contractions, depending on the intensity of the orgasm, which occur as close as 0.08 seconds apart. They are big old limiters in the Orgasm People's minds. They say M & J imposed the male's ejaculatory orgasm model on females, while actually, they say, women have the ability to experience multiple variations and degrees of orgasmic sensation far beyond men. And women would, if they only knew they could. The Orgasm People are on a mission to let everyone know the potential that's out there. "Expand your mind about the type of sensation you can have and value as pleasurable," Neil said.

So if I poke Clitty Rose and she feels a little bit good: I've had an orgasm. Seems almost like cheating. It's too easy. But I'll give her a whirl.

December 9, 11:15 p.m. PWCT

It didn't happen. I got distracted. As I went to masturbate, I heard some rumblings in the kitchen and I had to go see what was going on. My co-camper was there with a two-liter bottle of wine, beads of sweat on his forehead. He offered me a glass; I couldn't refuse. We got to talking. As he guzzled, he started in on a sad commentary on his life. It was a narrative of bummerdom. He said he was taught that he'd go blind and grow hairy hands if he ever touched himself; he still hadn't freed himself from his anxiety about self-loving. Sex was the toughest stuff in his life. He seemed more troubled by it than by death.

He said his wife had pleasure anxiety too. "I look at how happy all these women are here," he said, "and . . ." He put his hands through his white hair and stared into space. Our conversation ended with his face in his hands. He groaned, "I miss sex with my wife."

I had a weird experience looking at a grown man like that, utterly lost and utterly inconsolable. I shouldn't say it, I didn't say it, but I'll write it: He made me scared.

I don't want to end up like that.

I don't want anyone to end up like that.

December 10, 5 p.m. PWCT

I watched Samantha, who had been my original contact here, orgasm for an hour. The Orgasm People have a coming stage, an orgasm theater, in their basement. It has an electric-blue background with IKEA-looking white Chinese lanterns hanging around the perimeter. Samantha was up on a table with the whole family sitting around her as Neil strummed her clit. Wendy fed her water through a bendy straw. My co-camper looked on longingly. His fingers were twitching; I think they were enviously strumming an air-clit, keeping rhythm with Neil.

When my co-camper was moaning behind closed doors, hearing it seemed indecent. But Samantha was so out in the open now that everything seemed natural. If I could moan, I'd plagiarize Samantha. Those coming sounds should be copyrighted. Neil would be billed as the composer, I suppose.

Then I spoke up. "What does a dude get out of all this clit-rubbing?" I asked. All the dudes were doing was clit-rubbing. What about those blue balls they always complain about?

I thought Neil was going to take out his pocketknife again but use it on me this time. Instead he furrowed his brow.

"He gets a happy woman," he said. He said it like I should have known. "Producing a gigantic orgasm in a woman's body is the friendliest thing a man could do," he said. "A happy woman makes a happy man."

And just now, it looked like a happy woman made a happy room. All the women up on the stage straightened their backs, their cheeks flushed so much that they'd match their homemade raspberry preserves. Samantha was coming for everyone, and everyone felt it. "Good one, Samantha," said Eloisa with her eyes closed. "That was nice," said Wendy. "Nice peak," said Collin.

They were one big mass. They were a heap of personhood—not even skin was a boundary for them. Maybe those Craigslist sex prowlers I had interviewed months ago were actually more enlightened than I had given them credit for. Maybe an orgasm wasn't *owned*, because here it certainly wasn't anybody's possession: it was shared.

"You can wiggle your finger until the day you die," Neil said, noting that DOing can be a lifelong activity.

That's what my parents said about tennis. My parents were losing mojo by the minute here.

December 11, 11 a.m. PWCT

I was soon to head to the airport. The Orgasm People were running late for an interview we'd planned, so I milled about. I ran into Collin and tried not to think about DOing so he wouldn't think I wanted him to DO me, like maybe I did.

"Maybe I'll see you again sometime," Collin said.

I think he knew. He knew what I was thinking.

"Yeah, maybe so," I said.

I said it kind of flirty. My hand reached up and put a strand of hair behind my ear.

Then he said, "And maybe not."

And just like that he turned and walked away. I screwed up my face like I had eaten something sour. Then I shoved a banana into my mouth.

Time for the interview. Neil was in a big, blue terrycloth bathrobe, sipping coffee. The women surrounding him were already dressed and posture-perfect on the sofa.

Only a few minutes remained before I had to leave for the airport. Instead of letting me do the interviews like I wanted to, they chose to use that time to teach me a few things. They called sexual energy, or bodily energy in general, tumescence. They said you can use your tumescence in any way you want, but you are responsible for your own, and the most effective way to use it is through orgasm.

Basically, they told me, I'd been irresponsible with my tumescence and all weekend it had been overflowing from my body and into theirs. They had to do something with the excess and wound up having to do triple the usual DO sessions. That's why they were late. (Then I realized that it was true; they'd been running late for class all weekend.)

"You're saying I tumesced you guys?" I said. They laughed. I felt guilty. "Sorry," I said.

This was kind of awkward. It was like they'd been off-site masturbating me without me knowing. Everyone knew how pent-up and libidinously jammed I was.

"You've learned to be pretty civilized with it," said Neil. "It leaks out, you know. You blurt out sometimes, but overall, you're pretty civilized."

I tried to make excuses for why I was so sexually retrograde, bringing up all the things I thought were the culprits: Bangkok, Keena, creepy Baskin-Robbins guy, society . . .

Neil interrupted, telling me that victims, despite society's view on the issue, are not heroes. "It's easy to play victim," he said, "because then you don't have to take responsibility."

I looked at the women; they were all nodding in agreement.

"It could take you a lifetime to untangle all that shit," Neil said. "Meanwhile you could be going toward what you want."

It was time for me to go back to New York.

PART IV

THE CASE OF THE MISSING MEMOS

New York was the same save for the mid-December drop in temperature, but I'd changed. So people said. My mom said I sounded grounded. Leigh said something looked different about me—maybe my cheeks were rosier or I laughed easier. When I passed Atman at the Greenmarket, he touched my hand and looked me straight in the eyes. "Something very healthy happened to you while you were away," he said. "Lots of healthy stuff." He looked away before he saw my confirming smile.

But it was hard for me to believe that my little crotch sneeze had actually changed me. I didn't feel much different, but maybe I was. I got along with the cats a little better. I even found myself knocking a lamp chain back and forth like one of the pussies would a string, but maybe it's not such a good sign to get along with an animal that has a brain the size of a one-serving pudding. For what it's worth, I had lost my father's dissertation. I realized it one night when I had trouble sleeping and went looking for it. Maybe that meant that over the month away, I had become a little less fettered by my upbringing (sorry, Dad).

I was supposed to move forward now and take responsibility, as the Orgasm People had told me, but all I did was look backward. I riffled through my shelves, upturning stacks of old mail and magazines to find the sleeping mask Joe had left behind several months ago. I whiffed it. His pungency was gone; it smelled like my room now. It was over.

A lot of things had me thinking about Joe, and about relationships. There was going back to work at the bar, where every human outpost seemed to either be an amalgam of four legs, two torsos, and two lips—or trying to be. They all made connecting look so easy, so natural.

Then, when I called my grandparents, they wanted to know if I'd moved on to the *Gone With the Wind* portion of my book yet, meaning to ask, I believe, whether there were any romances—torrid or otherwise—that would lead to great-grandchildren. They didn't even ask me about my orgasm. And then there was Leigh, who was distraught that she was heading into her mid-thirties still single. "I want to be in love," she said. "I want to have someone who takes me out to dinner and wants to take care of me." When she said that, I couldn't say it didn't strike a chord somewhere in my underbelly, but I won't say it did, either.

So after extricating Joe's sleeping mask, I had the urge to throw it onto The Collector's jumble of junk, which had grown to a nice, even layer of trash bags while I was gone. But I didn't. I tucked it back behind some books on my shelf. A souvenir is a souvenir—you've got to save them.

I had my first visit with Rori since coming back. Maybe she had worried that I'd cured myself while I was away because she had planted a *Cosmopolitan* magazine in the waiting room, as if to ensure her three o'clock slot remained full by further ruining my psychology. By the time I flipped through the magazine, there wasn't one thing that was right with me. A-holes.

Rori was still on her Diet Peach Snapple kick. You'd think she'd go for some hot tea or at least something a tinge more wintery.

I'd been looking forward to this appointment for weeks. I dove right in. I didn't even have to chew my cheek this time around; it was already so thoroughly knotted from the past month that it had become a permanent fixture with perfectly grooved marks for my teeth to rest on.

"I don't think I got the memos," I began.

Rori leaned forward. She put her hands together. "What memos?" she asked.

"All the memos that tell you the stuff you're supposed to know," I said.

"Like which ones?"

"Well, I obviously didn't get the orgasm memo," I said.

"What else?"

I told her about all the people in the bar, coupled up.

"I didn't get the how-to-have-a-relationship memo or the settling-down memo."

"Any other memos?"

"All the memos," I said. "I think someone's blocked my memos."

She ran her fingers through her hair. She took a sip of Snapple.

"How can you know about all the memos," she asked, "if you're not getting the memos?"

I had to give it to her for that: That was a good point. She said I must be throwing away the memos.

"Why are you avoiding the memos?"

I shrugged.

"Come on, take a guess."

I shrugged again.

"Maybe it's a way to avoid rules," she said. Then she brought up my earlier talk about how I'm a bit envious that cats or even people who have lost—or never even had—their faculties (the intellectually disabled is a reference that I often make, she noted) get to act emotionally delinquent without repercussion. I think she was insinuating that I was losing my memos on purpose, losing them so I could act retarded too.

I started shaking my head. I was opposed to her breaking my reality. Why did she talk so much? I thought therapists were supposed to appear interested and pretend to listen. And really, why was she still drinking Diet Snapple? Snapple was so nineties. Why was I depending on someone who drank Snapple to help me shape my experiences in the twenty-first century?

As I left the building, I tried to access my memos. Maybe I'd unconsciously flagged all memos to be heaped into the spam lobe of my brain.

WHEN THE UNCOMPLICATED
BECOMES COMPLICATED

Avoiding? I wasn't avoiding anything. I went back to OneTaste to prove it to myself. I paid $250 for an introductory OMing (Orgasmic Meditation) course. I was going to take my pants off.

After a lot of New Age talk about orgasms allowing you to realize your true purpose, we finally got to try OMing. It wasn't mandatory, but the Orgasm People said I should go toward what I want, and I wanted to want the OneTaste lifestyle. They were liberated. They explored. They found meaning. They were researchers. They questioned society's strictures. And hey, they had orgasms every day. I could be like that. So I lay down.

Unfortunately, I didn't have an orgasm—not even by OP standards. My clit went numb again—it had stage fright—which wasn't surprising, considering the circumstances.

Everything about this didn't feel right. We rolled out yoga mats on the wood flooring. They were about a foot apart, twenty of them. From wall to wall, the apartment was crammed with people. Pants came off. Legs spread apart.

As I waited for my first OM to begin, I gazed at my ant tattoo; it didn't help calm me. Picking at my head bump just worried me—maybe it's cancer.

"It's *just* sex," someone said to quell me.

Just sex. *Just* sex. Just SEX. Just SEX.

A stranger was my partner. He had the job of rubbing the upper left-hand quadrant of my clit for fifteen minutes with his index finger. He had to rub out the "static" energy, which they say gets locked in the genitals from an accumulation of neglected desires.

Mind you, we had no liquor to temper any of this vividness. This was vivid stuff. I felt vivid. I was in a room full of naked about-to-be-throbbing beavers. I felt none of the serenity I'd felt at the Orgasm People's ranch.

The teacher, who was in his mid-twenties with a shaved head, became a drill sergeant. It was a completely sterile atmosphere. No romance was involved in this orgasmic exchange. Orgasm became a gym exercise. He pressed his stopwatch. "Stroke," he commanded.

He paced up and down the room.

"Make noises, ladies!" he screamed.

Moans happened all around me. I rolled my head to the side and all I could see were engorged lips—of both kinds—everywhere.

"Here's your clit," my partner said, twittering his index finger.

I was glad he had located it because I was laughing too hysterically to feel anything.

"Laughing is a defense mechanism that blocks pleasure," I was told by an instructor.

What if I didn't want what I thought I wanted? I wanted to want it, but maybe it wasn't a desire after all. Maybe women *are* sensually deprived, as OneTaste preaches—I could agree with that—

but I didn't want to be restocked in a long lineup of twats, getting stroked by a stranger.

"Can you feel it?" shouted the teacher, pacing the room with his stopwatch. "Go faster. Stroke like a little hummingbird."

The words "orgasm Nazi" came to mind as the teacher crouched near my partner. He looked into my legs like he was a miner, employed to oversee a cave with negligible coal production. "Stroke," he said. "Fast and light. Fast and light. Fast and light."

As soon as he said, "Time," I yanked up my pants. But before I charged out of there, I hugged the people and said it was great and that I'd loved it. I was a fake. I was a fraud. "I'll be back to OM soon," I said. A phony. I couldn't reconcile not liking it, though. The practice was all about orgasm, and I was all about orgasm, right? I had to keep up appearances so I wouldn't confuse myself. Besides, I still wanted to interview The Gasm. I still wanted to ask her what the MEANING OF ORGASM was. Then I charged out the door, feeling like I had the beginnings of PTSD: Pussy Traumatic Stress Disorder.

When I got outside, my stroking partner was already out there rolling a cigarette. He gave me a what-the-fuck-was-that face, and I hit him with a ditto. We went to a nearby bar called O'Neils.

"I don't get it," he said. "Separate love and sex? Why?"

He asked the question I'd had trouble verbalizing lately.

Greg was in his thirties. He had a medium build and bright big eyes, and he wore a beanie as he sipped cabernet. That was his first time at OneTaste. He couldn't understand why all the focus was on the woman's genitals and orgasm.

"Women are sensually deprived," I said, echoing the teachings.

"I disagree," he said. "Women get to wear makeup, high heels. They can cry. They can take baths with bubbles. If a guy takes a bath with bubbles, he is immediately not manly."

WHEN THE UNCOMPLICATED BECOMES COMPLICATED

He said that when he was younger he had had a terribly traumatic moment when he was masturbating to a *Hustler* magazine and his mom caught him. She invited his sisters in to see how horrible their brother was, how horrible men were.

"Men grow up with a terrible chip on their shoulder," he said. "We're programmed to be a certain way, not to be sensitive, and also have a lot of shame for being male. We learn that we're needy of women, but at the same time we're dominant, scary, gross figures for them."

He said men should be men, but be in touch with their feminine side, which was different from being feminine. The best lovemaking he had ever had, he said, was when he envisioned himself making love like a woman. "It sounds weird," he said, "but I rubbed my pussy against her pussy, my breasts against her breasts; it was so much more full body. It didn't have to be all about my cock being hard."

He asked me why I was in the course. I told him I didn't know anymore.

I was soon at the bar again, serving enough gin and tonics to make an elephant belligerent. I served a man a cocktail while he was talking to a friend. He said men were so simple; all they need to be happy is something to stick their dick in. I'd just had my talk with Greg, and I now felt like everyone is complicated—advertising shallowness was simply a cop-out. "All men need is sex," the man said again. "Enough sex and we're happy." Shove your simplicity, your fallacious uncomplicatedness, up your ass, I thought, and think a little deeper, please: everyone is three-dimensional. That was my last day working at the bar. I only had three weeks before I was headed to Israel anyway.

TRIBUTARIES

"Orgasm cookies," said Dr. Komisaruk, the orgasm researcher. "I made them myself." He handed me a sparkly gift bag filled to the brim with chocolate-chunked goodies over the table of the sports bar we'd chosen to eat at on Christmas Day. I took a bite. He kept amazing me—neuroscientists can bake! We hadn't seen each other since the sex conference, so I quickly updated him on my orgasm; I told him that I'd had one. I explained that so far they were kind of unreliable, but assured him, a bit jokingly, that my eargasms were still working like clockwork.

"I stick that Q-tip in," I said, "and know I'll have a shudder down my spine. Why aren't crotch ones that easy?"

Instead of laughing along, Dr. Komisaruk became quite serious and began lecturing me about the vagus nerve that he and his colleague Beverly Whipple have deeply studied. Through their fMRI research, they found that women with severed spinal chords (the part that was traditionally thought to relay sensational crotch information to the brain) can still reach orgasm. He gives credit to the vagus nerve, which bypasses the spinal pathway. He said the vagus nerve goes from the cervix through the viscera and all the way to the brain, connecting at the medulla oblongata.

"But what does that have to do with my easy eargasm?"

"Hold on," he said.

I was always interrupting. He was always telling me to hold on.

He said that the vagus has several branches, like tributaries, that flow into the nerve's main trunk. One such tributary becomes shallow at only one location on the body: the ear. He said no eargasm studies existed yet, but he believed it was possible that my eargasm was a valid orgasm caused by the Q-tip stimulating the very neural pathway that transports cervical orgasms. My ear sensations were riding the very legitimate vagus orgasm track!

Dr. Komisaruk smiled big and crammed a stuffed potato skin down his maw. As he chewed his eyes got really bright and I could see he was developing a plan. Orgasm, especially new orgasm ideas, really excited him, like when he realized he could preserve grant money by fashioning his own dildos, which his subjects used during experiments. He'd cut and polish Plexiglas rods and then use dental adhesive to secure a modified tampon to the top. Instead of paying $60 a pop at the sex toy stores, his handmade dildos cost him only a dollar apiece. When he finally finished swallowing, he said he wanted me to Q-tip myself in an fMRI to see if my eargasm turned on the same parts of the brain that a typical orgasm would. We could perform the first eargasm study and prove its existence in a tangible way! But then, suddenly, his face grew rather dim when he realized a problem. He said that as it stands, unfortunately, there was no space for Q-tipping, especially the Q-tipping I like to do, in the fMRI machine they use. Once the head is in there, there's basically only enough room to blink. I was still excited though. Dr. Komisaruk had made my eargasm sound no less important than any other type of gasm. He totally held an equal-opportunity stance for the gasms.

Then I asked how the other fMRI work was coming along and if I'd be able to participate in the study, especially now that I kind of sort of had my orgasm. He said he was still filling out more grant applications. He couldn't have looked less surprised, nor I, as he told me that nothing had come through yet.

Insert society-does-not-value-pleasure quote here.

Pleasure wasn't all he was concerned with, though. He had also found that orgasm might hold the answer to his lifelong goal: to find out how consciousness is formed from neurons. He said the answer might lie in the climax. With his fMRI orgasm scans, he could see how neurons spark and interact. "The activity of those neurons is somehow generating the conscious experience," he said, "so I'm still getting to it. I haven't given up on a damn thing!"

We continued eating the greasy potato skins as he tried to talk over some sports game playing loudly on the television. He said he was writing a chapter about consciousness for a book: "I'm calling the chapter 'Where Is I?'"

"Where is I?" I asked. "That's a great question."

"Where is I?" he shouted proudly.

"So, where is I?" I asked.

"We don't know where the 'I' is yet," he explained.

He said he hoped the fMRI would be approved soon so that he could use my neurons to continue the search for the origins of the first person singular. I told him I knew a lot of people who spent thousands of dollars trying to find themselves—their "I"—in all sorts of far-off locations or by going to self-help conventions, so I was sure there'd be a lot of interest if he found out that the "I" might actually be much closer to home.

THE PUSSY WHISPERER MAKES HIS
SOPHOMORE APPEARANCE

As I run around Prospect Park, I usually think about banging: proper banging, inadequate banging, self-banging, other people's banging, once-upon-a-time banging, and even happily-ever-after banging. But as I ran around the park this time, I wondered why Rori had suggested that I start having sessions twice a week.

All I did was tell her about those eye floaters I had, about the little cobweb-like strands that I saw when I looked into the sky. I told her that each little strand looked like it was on fire and running about, haywire. "It's all sparkly like that sometimes," I'd said. My floaters were out of control.

"Maybe they're tears that you're holding back," she'd said. Then she said, "You know, why don't you come in twice a week?" and gave me this face so sad I wanted to cradle it.

Was I *that* messed up?

As I left, I concocted a new suspicion: maybe Rori was a lesbian and wanted to date me. With an extra hour a week, she could woo me, but then again, maybe *I* was the lesbian and had a crush on her. And I know about transference, the phenomenon of redirecting feelings for one person to another unconsciously, but this wasn't transference, because whom did I feel that way toward? Maybe I should ask her out to coffee, a Snapple? I could learn to embrace the Snapple. We could make a cute but quirky love story. It happened in movies all the time—therapist and client. We'd be life imitating art, or at least pop culture. But it wouldn't work out, we'd get sick of each other, fawning, festering, falling apart. Then who would be there to tell me I didn't cry enough?

I'd told her I thought we should stick with one session per week.

I needed to get back to basics. That's what I decided as I finished my run around the park. This whole quest was about orgasm, and I hadn't been orgasming much since that first one in San Francisco.

So I went home and plugged in my vibrator. For the next few days, I holed up in my room. I had crotch sneeze after crotch sneeze. These orgasms were nice, but they weren't so impressive. Okay, why lie? They were actually pathetic. Sexologists I spoke to said it was all about building the proper neuro-passageways. These passageways need to be cleared and then paved with lots of feedback loops—that meant I needed to be having more orgasms. I was late to the game, so I had to work even harder. But I didn't have the patience to relax and breathe. I kept barely squeezing these comes out, going over the top with a scrunched-up face like I was climax-constipated.

Eric, my sacred whore, had been sending me instant messages lately. Often a variation of:

Eric: /appear! /pounce! /massage! /pleasure! /disappear!

I didn't respond right away because I felt a little awkward about having a sacred whore, but I figured he'd probably be the right person to take my orgasm to the next level. No dependency there, just

THE PUSSY WHISPERER MAKES HIS SOPHOMORE APPEARANCE

a good, honest masturbatory education. I did as a girl does when she has questions: I went to my crotch guru. The whole way there, I cursed my desire to always seek answers from others.

The vegetables were looking their illest during this late December. There were a few final piles of squash—the last zucchinis of the season—but none worth Kegeling about. The wind was whipping, but Atman, as always, was smiling.

"Beautiful day," he said, as I watched paper coffee cups and newspaper pages flip wildly on the asphalt. Pedestrians held gloved hands to shield their faces.

"Hmmm," I said. "I guess so, sure."

"What is it, sweetie?" he asked, as he took my hands and kissed them both. "How is the babe inside?"

His disciples, who help with sales, flanked him, so attempting privacy, I quietly told him I'd been thinking a lot about intimacy and relationships.

"When the time come," he said, "somebody gonna come equal to your own level."

"When?" I said, excited. "When will I find that somebody?" I always forgot Atman wasn't a fortune-teller and that I wasn't looking for anybody anyway. That was just me on auto-pilot.

"You know the soul inside," he said, pointing toward my heart. "And you know the libidic body," he said, gently shaking my shoulders. "This is a casually occupied vehicle to walk and breathe, to make the momentum. So you're not going to blame if you have sexual intimacy if he's not at the state of mind you're walking, breathing."

His use of language was sometimes so obscure, almost his own distinctive poetry. I think he was telling me to get some action already, telling me to call up my sacred whore immediately. That's how I interpreted it, anyway.

"My matter is you don't trust her," he said. "You talk to friends, you go to the library, but she is the master."

He was pointing at Clitty Rose, at my flower.

I picked up some baked goods—two raisin scones—and paid him.

"Make sure not to get a sickness, you know," he said, still pointing to my crotch. "That's not her kind, she's very picky in that sense."

"No kidding," I said.

"She's very picky in that sense," he repeated. "It's a little bit neurological with your psychology."

Atman hugged me, and as I walked away, he shouted out a last piece of advice, a loud piece of advice that anyone could hear.

"Remember," he called after me, bobbing his head. "Belly-button, tits, earlobes—those energies, the flower will open very widely." He opened his palm to the sky. "Waaah!"

A colorful sheet with an Indian print was beneath me, growing vibrant and dark again with each candle flicker. A CD compilation of African women singers hummed softly on my stereo. Earl the Stuffed Elephant was kicked off earlier. Pillows propped up my neck comfortably. I looked toward my toes. My legs were spread. Eric, my sacred whore, was between them, sitting on his knees.

"We're going to have lesbian sex," he said. "This is how lesbians have sex every night; they're doing it all over the world right now!"

He had a large purple vibrator he called the Saber in one hand and a very veiny hot-pink dildo in the other. "This is the kind I like to explore my ass with," he said, smiling as he wiggled the phallus in the air.

This moment wasn't occurring instantaneously; it had taken three hours of coddling to get there. We started by having dinner. It was the first time I had seen Eric outside of the Temple of Betty.

THE PUSSY WHISPERER MAKES HIS SOPHOMORE APPEARANCE

He seemed awkward. While in the restaurant, he was as out of place as a cowboy at the Ritz Carlton, but once we got back to my place and he spied the bed in my room, it was like he was back on his horse. It was my turn to freeze up.

Eric stripped down to his sex professional workout gear—that same quick-dry spandex shirt he had worn before—but still had on his black jeans. He looked at himself in my full-length mirror. "If I was gay," he said, "I'd fuck me." I cringed. He said it loud. My roommate, Leigh, shares a wall with me, and I'm sure she heard him. If he was a date and not my sacred whore—sacred whores have much more behavioral leeway, I've found—I'd have kicked him out immediately. But the way he said it, come to think about it, was actually endearing, because I knew he meant it. If he *were* gay, he would figure out a way to penetrate himself. I'm sure of it.

I tried to quiet him, but he was really into the subject at hand. Eric said he'd always wanted to get physically fit to the point where he'd want to fuck himself; it took him a long time to get there. He explained the book, *The Orgasmic Diet*, which helped him. He said Marrena Lindberg, the author, was chubby, so it wasn't a weight-loss kind of thing, but more of a get-your-*grrr* type endeavor. Omega-3 tablets, take four a day, Eric said. Lots of steamed vegetables. No white bread. No smoking. That's like poison to the orgasm, he said. And absolutely no soy. "I love soy," I said. "No soy!" he reiterated. Memory would get clearer, and when the body and brain were functioning optimally, they could react better to stimuli. "The better your orgasm is," he said, "the healthier you'll know you are."

"Now that you have your orgasm," he continued, "we have to worry about increasing the strength. We want your eyes to roll back and for you to bang your head against the mattress because it's so good." He feigned falling backward; I could see the whites of his eyes.

He began massaging me. My clothes came off very slowly. He told me about a way of touching someone called "the taking touch." It's when you touch the other person in the way that feels best to you, and because it feels right for you and you are engaged in it completely and confidently, it should feel right for the other person. If that's what he was doing, then it's true: it felt amazing.

I was a vehicle. He was a mechanic. He knew about all my levers and pulleys. He was trying to rev me, getting me in the right gear by pressing all my buttons.

"Can I go down on her?"

He was talking about my nipple.

When I started to shimmy away, he said, "Pleasure reluctance." That became his refrain for the evening. He said pleasure reluctance was natural, and I had to break through it by breathing.

I couldn't hear the music anymore over my shouting. He'd grabbed my feet and shoved each little digit in his mouth. I was shouting warnings at him.

"Pleasure reluctance," he said.

"No, beware," I said. "I have toe jam."

At least with Fred the foot fetish man, I'd washed them.

"I wouldn't do anything I don't want to," he said.

It'd be nice if no one did anything they didn't want to; then I wouldn't have to always waste my time worrying if they were liking it or not. But this was lunacy; this was a health risk. I looked on in disbelief as he wove his tongue in and out of every dip, every crevice, every surface of my hoof. I'm no pedicure girl either, not even close. You couldn't pay me to put my feet in my mouth—I know where they've been—but Eric looked even more nourished than when he had been eating sushi earlier in the evening.

THE PUSSY WHISPERER MAKES HIS SOPHOMORE APPEARANCE

I felt a big case of pleasure reluctance rising and a desire to hide in the bathroom; I tried to sublimate with inhalation. That's what's awful about sacred whore sessions at your own apartment; you can't run away. You're there. You're stuck. Or maybe it's a good thing—it's the only way I'd stay.

All of a sudden he was everywhere at once.

"Your tits have nice resistance," he said, cupping them. "They're thick." I'd never been called thick and taken it as a compliment, but coming from Eric, it sounded like all tits should be thick.

He caressed me and started making little barking sounds, like a sea lion pup. He said it was a man's job to fight his *grrr* with sensitivity. "Most men push, poke, and pull," he said, tracing circles around my nipple. "Not good." Moments from my past came to mind when I thought I might suffer a spontaneous mastectomy due to some man's overzealous paws. They're not screw tops; they don't come off. Eric's face suddenly lit up as he began to softly knead my breast. "It feels like I'm moving my fingers over rows and rows of a well-gardened plot of land," he said. "It goes in a spiral that ends in a nice little nugget at the top."

I grinned and unfortunately thought of my parents' nursery. I bet they'd be proud to know that there was at least an essence of a good gardener somewhere inside me.

This was when Eric brought out a sparkly, fuchsia-colored gift bag. "Some things to try," he said. "If we want to."

The contents—a dildo, a vibrator, and lubricant—now sat before him. These items made my little plug-in look like novice stuff. That vibrator was a baby. I asked if he was jealous about all the toys women could use. He said he was jealous they had more slots to put toys into, but he had his penis, which he called a big clitoris, that he could use to insert, so he wasn't really all that jealous. He called it even. He said there were a lot of dyke women who were envious of his big clitoris; they'd love to be able to feel their girl-friend's insides with their little clits. So he was happy he could feel the insides of the girls he liked.

He handed me the Saber and said I'd be in charge of clit stim. (I guess the whole word, stimulation, is too hard to say if you're using it nine hundred times a day.) To get started, he'd control the dildo portion of our lesbian sex.

I looked down and saw him between my legs, sitting with perfect posture and the fluorescent phallus resting by his hip. I got up on my elbows and started inching backward.

"Pleasure reluctance," he said.

I plopped back down.

He gandered directly into my vulva. I was still seeing him like a mechanic—a mechanic consulting on my orgasm gear. He was used to this crotch stuff. I didn't have to be nervous. I didn't have to worry about him looking at or wanting to play with other vulvas—like I would have if he were a romantic interest—because I already knew he'd been playing with tons. Vulva was his career.

He slipped his thumb in and then he told me to tighten and release—engaging in the Kegel motion. He was warming me up for the big pink thing. It took a while and required some deep concentration on my part not to clamp down while he got it in there. The insertion portion wasn't particularly pleasing. "Now clit stim," he ordered. He yanked the Saber from me, notched it up until it was shaking real good, and passed it back like it was a lollipop. I plunked it on top of my clit. "Don't keep it still," he said softly. "Move it back and forth."

He was sliding the dildo in and out, gently. Real good. Real often. Every three seconds or so, he'd plunge it in again. I started thinking of him as a plumber, plunging for my orgasm. I believed in him: I knew he'd unclog that sucker.

THE PUSSY WHISPERER MAKES HIS SOPHOMORE APPEARANCE

"Why'd you stop?" he asked.

I'd lost track of my duties. One tool up in that area, you know, is a lot. My pussy had to be kind of surprised; she'd never had plastic—and definitely not hot pink—up there like that before.

"Pleasure reluctance," he said, so I breathed.

Then he told me to try both at once because he wouldn't be there every day for dildo duty. "It's best when you blend sensation," he said, "and get the clit on both ends. But it takes practice." I commandeered the dildo with the right hand and had the Saber in the left—it was like trying to pat your head and rub your belly. I was trying to hump with the vibrator and tickle with the dildo. Eric went mutiny-style and took back authority of the dildo. Maybe we were getting ahead of ourselves, he said.

We finally got some rhythm going. We were both succeeding at our respective tasks. We were both pumping the plastic back and forth. He said he loved his life. "Do you love yours?" he asked.

I looked down at Clitty Rose, at my cleft full of devices, and I thought for a second. "Yes, yes I do," I said. And then it started happening. The sensations became immense, or were they intense . . . no, these sensations were incoherent. They were a mess. They were happening in my clit, but they felt everywhere at once. I was trying to have the "right" kind of gasm—let the energy build naturally, not like the volcanic crotch sneezes I'd been having—but I started heating up like an overworked engine. We'd been going for about twenty minutes at least. I was hot, really hot, and dewy in all my gorges. I wanted to go into rigor mortis, I wanted to make all those muscles tighten and pop one out, but no. I didn't want to look like a dead person in front of my sacred whore, especially now that I'd just told him how I love life. I stopped with the Saber; I couldn't do it anymore. I felt like the pads of my feet were on fire and wondered what kind of weird neural pathways I was building. I wasn't sure I wanted to be building those.

Eric stopped. He gently pulled out the dildo. "I love that suction sound," he said. I personally thought it wasn't much more pleasant than nails on a chalkboard. I was kind of disappointed; I'd expected it to happen.

"Did it feel good?" he asked, cuddling next to me.

"I didn't orgasm," I said.

"But did it feel good?" he said.

"Really good," I said.

"Then perfect."

He told me I'd come a long way since our last session, since he'd introduced me to me and determined my scent was a twinkle. "The twinkle doesn't last forever," he said. That sounded like a warning.

While he showered off, I leaned out my window, breathing in the cold air and letting myself (also my soles) simmer down. When I was with a guy like Eric—so patient and sensitive—he made me believe there was no way the whole gender couldn't totally love and respect every cunt out there.

Eric walked in. "I get it!" I shouted. "I finally get it: men really do love women!"

I half-expected him to get naked, maybe even jack off to the excitement of my discovery, but instead he looked concerned.

"*Some* men really love women," he said. "Some. Be careful."

I let Eric out, but he left the goodies for me to experiment with. As I heard him creaking down the stairs, I was amazed at my lack of romantic feelings. Eric was both business and pleasure, and somehow I'd really done a topnotch job of not leaking out one drop of sentimental emotion about the whole ordeal.

I went back to my room to put myself over the top. My orgasm must have been afraid of other people because I undid that friction right fast.

THE PUSSY WHISPERER MAKES HIS SOPHOMORE APPEARANCE

I called Fiona after I finished. She was in San Diego visiting her family for the holidays. She thanked me for the vulva ring. I'd sent it to her for Christmas. She said it created a real awkward moment around the Christmas tree. She said everyone passed it around in silence until her dad finally said something so they could all get on with it.

"Now you have two," he'd said.

I thought that was funny.

Then I told her I was worried that I was going to start decorating my house with dildos like many of the other sex people I had met. I told her to slap me really hard if she found a dildo mobile hanging above my bed next time she came over.

I went on to explain what Eric and I had done that evening. I thought I'd be ahead of her on this one; not even she could have gotten this memo.

"He called it lesbian sex," I said. "Two toys at once. Isn't that craaaazy?"

"I don't know, Mara," she said. "I think everyone does that. I do it."

"What the fuck," I said. "Who taught you that?"

And she just giggled. "It's great, right?"

MANDATORY

MASTURBATION

INTERMISSION

THE SEXTH SENSE

I don't know what it is, but the Orgasm People must have some sort of otherworldly orgasm perception. They were kind of freaking me out; they sensed my orgasmic status even when I was clear across the continent. Samantha called me the day after I saw Eric.

"Do you have any research partners yet?" she asked.

I started to describe what had happened with Eric. "He brought me these amazing toys and . . ."

"Vibrators?" she said, with a cautionary sharpness in her tone.

"Yes," I squeaked. "What'd I do wrong?"

"A vibrator can be a quick jerk-off," she said. "Don't get seduced by it. With vibration and pressure, women get more and more numb over time. They have to go faster and faster in order to get one, and then they get a big release because the body is so starved for orgasm, but the genitals are getting number."

"No vibrators?" I asked. I was befuddled. I never realized the Orgasm People didn't believe in toys.

"It doesn't promote engorgement or intimacy with another person," she said. "It limits how much fun you can have. You have a lot of education and information and you'll make the right choice. Exploit sensation, feel more, and have more."

One sex person tells me to use vibrators, other sex people say no. All of a sudden I felt very behind. What to do?

I had to leave for Israel in a couple days anyway. I told Samantha I was going away and she said she wanted to keep in touch to help me get back on track; she'd call me when I returned.

When I came out into the living room, Ursula was working on her documentary and Leigh was drinking a tea with soy, which I had learned the night before was anti-orgasm liquid. I didn't chide her for fogging her orgasm, but I did whip out my two new toys, shove them probably a little too close to their faces, and ask what they thought of them.

Turns out I wasn't the only one who hadn't gotten the lesbian sex memo. I felt a lot better knowing that other people hadn't, either, but I felt bad that Leigh had to spit up her tea like that, even if it was better for her orgasm.

Later that day, Leigh and I went out to dinner. She said something that got me in a tizzy. It really did. "You don't have to become an expert," she said. "Just a few months ago you were new to all this and now you're with professionals. You don't have to get your black belt."

I told her I liked what I was doing. I was learning a lot.

"What about your heart?" she said. "I'm worried about your heart."

So of course after she said that, I too started worrying about my heart. I'm a preventative hypochondriac, you know. I worry about things before I have the symptoms so that I don't have to be in pain, but she made me realize that in this case the symptoms were already present: I could no longer feel anything.

But there was no time to worry about it now. Israel was right around the corner, and I hadn't prepared anything yet. I got going. I visited the dermatologist because I feared that the head bump I was constantly picking was cancerous. The Holy Land has historically been a popular place to die, but I wasn't ready for that kind of commitment.

The cancer was actually a wart. The doctor froze it off.

Conclusion: I'm disgusting.

Post-conclusion: What am I supposed to pick at now?

I told Atman I was leaving. "This is the proper time," he said. "You have to mature yourself, that's the best way."

"Are you calling me a late bloomer?"

"Not bloomer," he said. "Flower, sweetheart. It's your flower."

The day before I left, Leigh came out of her room, waving a bundle of square aluminum packets. She was laughing hysterically, with a smile I wasn't sure was pleased or maniacal. "My condoms expired," she said, letting the sheet unfold like an accordion in her hands. "My condoms expired!"

Which made me wonder, how long had it been since I'd had actual man sex—not Tantric sex, not lesbian sex, not sacred whore sex, not me-on-me sex. I counted on my fingers and got up to my left-hand pointer finger: I was going on seven months now.

I should have realized how long it'd been. My recent actions were blatantly trying to let me know. After all, I had gone to a masquerade party for New Year's in a mask shaped like a hot dog in a bun. People were all too ready to let me know that I had weenie on the brain. And then there was Earl the Stuffed Elephant's trunk— I'll just say its choice of location when I woke up never ceased to surprise me.

The night before I left, Zola took me out to Casa Mono, a tapas bar specializing in just about everything unkosher. She took me just in case Israel gave me a big lazy-Jew spanking, like it had done to my brother. "This might be your one last chance for pig!" she said. She ordered something with lard and shellfish. We drank and ate up the proceeds of her last Tantra session—her client was a banker who wanted to be dressed up in panties, spanked, and then pissed on. "I'd NEVER drink piss," she said, "but to have *your* piss drunk, well, it's kind of amazing." She lifted her head toward the ceiling and mimicked her client, like a baby bird opening and closing its mouth, waiting for the mama bird to deliver the worm.

"Gross," I said.

"I think it's beautiful," she said, dropping a mussel into her yap. "We're all trying to satisfy ourselves," she said, pausing to moan as she swallowed the morsel. "He's lucky he found out how to satisfy himself."

SPIRITUAL GONORRHEA

My flight arrived at Ben Gurion International at five a.m. A big bald man named Shlomo "Momo" Lifshitz, the organizer of the trip, yelled, "Welcome home! Welcome home!" in a raspy baritone as hundreds of puffy-eyed Jews of the Diaspora schlepped to the baggage claim.

Since 2000, Jewish philanthropists have sent 190,000 Jews aged eighteen to twenty-six to visit Israel for their first time for the Birthright Project. Their hope is that we're still impressionable enough to develop a relationship with the place and that it will strengthen our Jewish identities. Some people I know call it propaganda, but I called it a free trip and the perfect opportunity to explore my orgasmic ancestry.

Tour guides loaded us onto buses—there were twenty-eight people on mine. We'd get no sleep before a full day of touring. Omer, a thirty-five-year-old Israeli man who would be our guide for the next ten days, took the bus mic. He wouldn't shut up. He had glasses and an unusual hairdo: a normal buzz cut until it reached his forehead, at which point he had strands cut straight across, not long enough to call bangs, not short enough to call anything else. "Here's an Arab village to your left," he said. "That's Jerusalem limestone to your right." He droned on nonstop; we couldn't even get one minute of sleep.

We stopped in Jerusalem's old city. In a haze from time-zone transplantation and the freezing winds careening down cobblestone streets, I focused maybe too much and too fast on my orgasm. I told Omer that I was writing a book and asked if during our trip he could point out anything orgasmic in nature or even, if he had a moment, some old whore temples. He seemed a bit creeped out.

"There are no whore temples," he said.

"No, I know they aren't active," I said. "But I read that there were temples like a couple thousand years ago with whores. You know, the sacred whores?"

He'd told us that he'd majored in history. So naturally, I thought he'd know. Maybe he was just playing ignorant, but he backed away slowly and told us to prepare notes to stick in the Western Wall (also called the Kotel), which was a remnant of the Holy Temple and therefore one of the holiest sites for Jews. He said we should leave a prayer to help us find our significant other.

"We are not whole in Jewish law by ourselves," he said. "We must find our other halves."

The Western Wall is partitioned—one side for men and the other for women. Women have about a third of the space; did that imply we actually had to find our significant other two-thirds? I wanted to say the disparity was because women are more petite, but unfortunately I couldn't convince myself of that, especially because the males seemed to get special treatment. Hasidic Jews with long beards, ear locks, and black hats urged the guys in the group to wrap leather straps called *tefillin* around their arms and head before saying a prayer. It looked like an interesting kind of bondage. The bondage wasn't for women. I finally had the desire to be roped up when it was forbidden.

I tore out a piece of notebook paper. I began to scrawl down a prayer. I did the best I could—nice and simple—given the sleep deprivation and my intermittent relationship with Judaism.

Dear W. Wall,
    Please deliver some pussy insight during my stay here and help me figure out what the *$%! my pussy wants. And if you have time, I heard my heart is worth worrying about.

Sincerely,
Mara Altman

(I didn't want to curse at the Wall.)

I crumpled my prayer up into a little ball—it looked like the spit wads kids used to blow through straws in elementary school—and lodged it deep into one of the crevices between the large stone blocks. All around me, women bobbed back and forth while reciting from the Torah. Men did the same on their side. Logan had told me that when I arrived, I'd feel like I'd found my people, and I didn't believe him until this moment. I thought it was weird at first—the people rocking—but then I realized they *were* my people because I started to see the rocking as humping: they were getting intimate with God!

As I adhered to convention by facing the Wall as I backpedaled out of there, I hoped it wasn't sacrilegious to pray for my pussy on such holy territory, but I figured it might actually be appreciated considering all the factoids I'd gathered about Judaism before I'd left New York City. I'd called up a rare breed of adviser: a rabbi sexologist from Los Angeles who had a particular interest in Kabbalah, Rabbi Ronald Levine.

SPIRITUAL GONORRHEA

I already knew Jews carry genetic diseases like Tay-Sachs and Crohn's, but I wanted to know if they had something more positive, like maybe a penchant for orgasms. After all, the Jew's first commandment is to be fruitful and multiply. Rabbi Levine told me female orgasm was an obligation for every Jewish husband. A woman who didn't get her orgasm had grounds for divorce. Not only that, but he said the Kabbalists, or Jewish mystics, believe the sexual satisfaction men give to women gratifies the Creator and helps keep universal harmony. Play with clits, not with bullet clips. "In Kabbalah," Levine said, "sex makes the world go round—God's world, your world. We're talking true pleasure here—not making kids—pure pleasure."

Conversely, Rabbi Levine was not every rabbi and conceded that the Torah was always interpreted differently. "During various periods of time and depending on which sources and eras you look at," he noted, "Judaism is not so nice about sexuality." So basically, like life, Jewgasmic potential was up to perception. In the following days, I'd have to decipher my own.

After several more stops—and a minute-by-minute narration by Omer—we finally made it to the hotel. Before we could go to sleep, we had one last discussion with Momo Lifshitz about our forthcoming journey. I wasn't expecting what he had to say: he basically told us to fuck, get fucked, or some combination of the two, but only do so if it was with a Jew. He told us the Jewish family was shrinking—only thirteen million now—and it was our responsibility to increase the number. That was quite a different message from Christianity and Buddhism, where the ideal devotee was a celibate monk, priest, or nun.

"Consider Birthright a matchmaking factory," he said. "The future of the Jewish family is in your hands. Open your eyes on a good opportunity. You arrived this morning, you're all good-

looking. Open your heart, open your arms, and find Jewish love."
He bribed us to hook up: he said if we found Jewish love on the trip
and got married, he'd bring us back for a free honeymoon.

I was tired, but I wasn't slow. I'd already scoped out everyone. I
checked out the women first to factor in my competition. I had us
all plotted on a graph in my head—big eyes, clear skin, corkscrew
curls, bubble ass, and thin all got a plus-one. But when I scoped
out the guys, I realized my plotting was a waste of time. None of
the men caught my attention. But I didn't completely shut out all
opportunities. I still harbored hope that I'd find someone who'd
collaborate with me on my orgasm. Besides it was, after all, only
day one.

A twenty-three-year-old woman named Rebecca and I became
friends. She scoffed at Momo's lecture; for her it wasn't all about
being fruitful and multiplying: she said it was all about finding
another woman. "Women know women," she said. "The soul connection is deeper." She was a Jewish lesbian.

There were all different kinds of Jews in Israel, not just the ste-
reotypical kind we have in the United States like lawyers, doctors,
and Hollywood folk. There were Jewish janitors, Jewish beggars,
bad Jews, tall Jews, ugly Jews, itty-bitty sweet Jews, even small-
nosed Jews, and, of course, Jewish bus drivers steering us around
the country. In the following days, we went to Haifa, Caesarea,
Akko, and Safed, an old Kabbalist town. While there, I asked Abraham, an artist-Kabbalist, if Kabbalah was synonymous with sex,
like what Rabbi Levine had said.

"I don't know what you're talking about," he said. Why did everyone feign ignorance? He seemed positioned to hit me over the
head with his credit card machine, which he used as everyone in
the group gathered to purchase souvenirs from his collection of
paintings.

SPIRITUAL GONORRHEA

"Kabbalah is life," he said scowling. Then he went back to swiping.

"In a way, isn't life sex?" I asked. He said nothing, probably because I had asked under my breath. I was afraid to get a Master-Card imprinted on my forehead. At least he didn't sell me a $2.50 bottle of special water like the Kabbalah Center in Manhattan had when I'd gone there to inquire. Instead, I bought a one-hundred-shekel print that I could point to as proof when I got home and say, "Hey, look, I was in Safed before!"

As the days went on, manly prospects diminished substantially. My mom had always told me I'd get along with Jew boys better; we'd have something innately in common. My grandparents said it too. "Being Jewish, we all grow up on lox and cream cheese in the same way," my grandpa said.

But despite what my family had to say, upon my Jewish awakening, I realized that a group of twenty-something male Jews was no different from any other group of twenty-something male humans. Our group regressed into something resembling a high school excursion. There was late-night drinking. I got to learn about—and luckily not experience—the shocker (when a guy sticks his fingers up a girl's pussy and ass at once), the superman (when a guy comes on a girl's back and then attaches a sheet so she has on a cape when the come dries), and the lovely acronym FUPA, for Fat Upper Pussy Area. Great, another fun thing to be insecure about.

Omer took his job seriously; when he wielded the microphone, he looked as proud as Poseidon holding his trident. Often when I asked a question, he'd say, "Mara, that's not relevant," and then he'd keep talking as I stood in the middle of some ruin, bewildered. The boys in the group called Omer the anti-poon. That was their way of saying he couldn't get pussy. It was very important for boys to determine who could and couldn't get pussy. Little did they realize that the more they discussed pussy as a commodity in front of the actual keepers of pussy, the less likely they'd be to get any.

Then my wallet disappeared—I didn't lose it; it disappeared. We were in Tiberias after all, close to the Sea of Galilee, where Jesus walked on water; strange phenomena obviously happened there. Everyone joined in the hunt for my money. We never found it. I tried to employ Omer to help me call my bank overseas. When I knocked on his hotel room door, he was busy watching a basketball game. He was my Judas, a complete jerk, and wouldn't tear his eyes from the screen. I wondered if what happened to me next had something to do with Mary Magdalene's hometown being only a few miles away, or if there were just so few male prospects in my vicinity, or maybe it was that wad I'd wedged into the W. Wall's crevice, but as he shut the door in my face, I had a searing sensation in my crotch. It was like the whole middle of me was dumped in a bucket of dry ice—it was so cold but so hot simultaneously.

Was Omer the Chosen One? The Jew who's supposed to collaborate with Clitty Rose for an orgasm?

After I spent an hour on the phone with the bank and an hour watching people get drunk, I retired to my bedroom and fantasized about being in Omer's room and making out with him during commercial breaks. I was sharing a room with Rebecca; she came in late. She woke me up. Her eyes were bugging out.

"What is this?" she said, pointing to her chin. "What is this?"

Her chin was chafed. It seemed the lesbian in the group was the only one getting any man action. She was trying to live up to her Jewish mission, but she wasn't privy to beard damage. She didn't know what stubble could do.

"I swear I'm staying gay the rest of my life," she said. I guess that's one way to keep your skin smooth.

SPIRITUAL GONORRHEA

As we moved north to the Golan Heights and then back down to Tel Aviv, Omer still had his boring moments, but I found myself more attentive. Even when he was droning, I was enraptured just by watching him point at a map, up and down along Israel's oblong-shaped territory.

He was dominating, impatient, and kind of an asshole, and he wore the same fleece every day. We'd never get along.

Is that why I wanted him so badly?

At the midway point of the trip, eight young Israeli soldiers joined our group. Here was our big chance to interact with our Israeli peers. Israeli soldiers, what were their orgasms like? I collected some stats on them. Verdict: very orgasmic except for one. He said he hadn't been able to come in six months, despite having sex, because life didn't matter anymore, nothing mattered anymore. "Now I know how women feel," he said.

Hmmm.

We charged down to the Bedouin tents in the Negev desert. We'd be staying with them for a night. There we could see how Muslims and Jews could be amicable toward one another. Oddly enough, the West Bank and Gaza weren't on the agenda for that. But I digress.

Camels meandered in front of the tents. We rode them. While up there on its hump, getting a camel toe of my own as my pants crept up, I asked my Jewish riding partner about sex. She said she loved orgasms, but not alone so much—the act of sex with another person gave her a feeling of self-worth.

The Bedouins demonstrated a traditional coffee ceremony, after which we could ask questions through a translator. My question about the effects of female genital circumcision was conveniently passed over. "Inappropriate," Omer chided me.

We were getting ready to go to dinner—a traditional Bedouin

feast where we could use our hands to stuff food into our faces. Omer was talking to me, Rebecca, and another girl. As he got up, he looked at me.

"Your eyes are an illusion," he said. "They aren't as big as they seemed."

"An illusion?" I said, transfixed.

"It's not that they're big," he said. "They're just what I see when I look at you."

"Why?"

"The color, I don't know."

I opened the door behind my eyes and let him in. "Maybe it's a thyroid problem," I said, trying to flirt.

He smiled. A laugh actually cracked on him.

He walked ahead of me. He had an olive complexion and broad shoulders that towered about a foot above my own. He sucked on a cigarette. I walked through the swirling smoke. It was forming undulating curlicues, almost like circles, which were kind of like Os—Big Os, I thought. I thanked W. Wall for supplying me with some tangible pussy insight, which was now just in front of me, sitting down to eat.

Rebecca saw my longing look. "Don't let it slip by," she said as she passed. Her chafe had turned into a dry patch by now.

The next day, we went to Masada, a fortress built by King Herod the Great. I caught up with Omer as we surfaced upon a plateau after hundreds of stairs took us upward. We could see for miles. The light brown ground met the blue sky at the horizon. Omer told us about a Jewish mass suicide that had taken place in the first century CE. "They'd rather die than come under Roman control," he said. When I looked at him, I didn't even see his weird haircut anymore. I noticed his full lips. There was a little crumb on the side; I wanted to lick it off. On the way down the mountain, he told me I needed a Hebrew name. He named me Noa. Noa means movement. My insides squirmed.

I'd become so intent on staring at Omer that I forgot I was trying to uncover my orgasmic roots. Ehud, a jewelry salesman, was helping tourists at his shop when I recalled my blunder. I engaged him in conversation.

"Only ten percent of ladies have orgasm, right?" he asked.

"No, many more have orgasm," I said, "but it's hard for them during sex."

"Then how do they get it," he asked, "like on a bike seat?"

"No, masturbation works," I said.

"Oh yes, masturbation."

"You think orgasm is important?" I asked.

"Fifty percent of the world is ladies," he said. "If all can have orgasm, they would be happier. With more happy, that would make the universe happier."

I liked his positive outlook, so I bought a pair of earrings from him. I could point to my earrings when I got home and say, "I got these near Masada where the Jews once killed themselves."

Then we went to Elat, a resort town near Egypt's border. We got ready for a night out, first dinner and then dancing. We went to Caldo Brazil, a Brazilian steak house. I wasn't hungry, but I was thirsty. There was red wine in my glass.

And then there wasn't.

My heart beat fast as we all strolled toward a bar called Unplugged. I walked with Omer. He told me the most precious thing the Jews have is Israel; it's worth fighting for, he said. I told him fighting wouldn't make anything better, but I was cynical. I had little belief the fighting would ever stop. I said the day there will be peace on Earth is the day we're faced with aliens, a common enemy to unite us. And then we will begin fighting in outer space.

But what I really wanted to say was that we'd heal the world faster if he began focusing on my crotch.

I didn't want the feeling in my groin to slip by. There were only two days left to make something happen, to finally experience this orgasm stuff with passion.

"There's something I actually wanted to tell you, and I hope you don't take it the wrong way or get offended, but . . ."

He looked at me. "Go ahead," he said.

"Um . . ." I said. "I'm really attracted to you. Really, really."

I suddenly felt like a two-year-old. He was a real Jew. I was a second-rater from the Diaspora. He'd been in the military. I'd told military recruiters on the phone to bugger off during dinner. He'd shot at people. I'd seen movies where people were shot at.

My heart was tripping.

"I'm a professional," he said. "I take my work seriously."

Shit. Fuck. I was about to be rejected. He had self-control; I could like him for that. In fact, Clitty Rose was buzzing now more than ever.

"I think you're special," he said.

I didn't want to know which kind of special he meant, so I didn't ask.

"I can't do anything until after the trip," he said, "but can I take you out to dinner after?"

"Uh-huh."

I didn't talk to him again that night until we all walked back to the hotel. I stood by him as everyone filtered inside.

We were alone outside. "Dear Noa," he said. "I must go to sleep."

He walked inside, and I didn't get to touch his lips. *If he looks back at me, he wants me bad.*

He didn't look back. Shit.

In the morning, I woke up with regret clouding my head more than my hangover. The pickled salmon at breakfast almost had me gagging. I saw Omer and said hi; he said hi back. The only acknowledgment of last night's discussion was a slight upturn of his lips, or was he just chewing?

Did all that actually happen?

When I got back to my room to pack up for our last two days in Jerusalem, I called the airline and extended my stay for four days. I had nothing to lose, except perhaps my belief in pussy awakenings and my dignity.

Each minute was like a countdown. My gut seared every time Omer picked up the microphone. Maybe even my heart was warming. I couldn't wait until everyone left me behind in the Holy Land and I could get my hands on his peninsula. There was no way something wouldn't happen. Something would happen.

Then something happened. We were on the bus. There was quiet—everyone was sleeping off the previous night's escapades—until I heard the rustle of a plastic bag somewhere near the front of the bus. Omer sat up there. Then I heard retching. A choking retch. Then more rustling and then a sigh.

Omer had thrown up.

Omer was violently ill.

Who's done this? W. Wall?

We went to Yad Vashem, the Holocaust memorial, on our final day. I felt so guilty while sitting through a talk given by a survivor because while he spoke about drinking another man's piss to survive, being separated from his family, being lashed twenty-five times on the ass because all he wanted was a turnip, I was thinking about giving Omer a wet willy with the tip of my tongue and hoping that he'd had proper female anatomical training. But things weren't looking good—Omer was the incarnation of an implosion, shuffling like someone had lit his asshole on fire. When he tried to muster a smile, the perspiration pooled on his forehead. My pussy was more confused than ever. She had found something she wanted, and it was about to keel over? There were still four days, I was sure he'd get better.

He had to get better.

No, really. He had to.

"How you feeling?" I asked him as I strolled by in the hall. He told me to stay in Tel Aviv during my remaining days. "I'll take you out tomorrow," he said breathlessly, as if he had a bullet wound in his abdomen.

I saw it already: We'd be side by side for four nights straight. I already had the shoes picked out he'd wear to break the glass on our wedding night. Jewish love! I'd get a free trip back!

Before heading back to the airport, to bring our journey full circle, we stopped one last time at the Western Wall. A woman held a mobile phone receiver up to the Wall so someone could make a long distance prayer. I thought she was cheating. I ripped off another piece of notebook paper. I felt much more focused than the time before.

I patted the stone. I felt like we—me and W. Wall—were old friends now. We'd been through a lot in the past ten days and I didn't want it to think I was ungrateful.

Dear W. Wall,

I want to thank you very much for making my pussy stir—if that was in fact you—but I'm a little perplexed. I mean, there are some mixed signals happening because the trigger to my

newfound arousal is currently upchucking in the men's stall. I
know you're probably very busy, but can we get that cleared up?
Again, thank you so much.

Sincerely,
Mara Altman

I wadded it up. It didn't stick in the crevice this time. I had to
keep bending down to pick it up and shove it back in. Then I subtly
rocked back and forth—I was still a little inhibited; not as comfortable as the other women—and I didn't want to be too obvious
about dry-humping the Creator in front of everyone.

There were lots of hugs at the airport. Lots of of-course-we're-all-
going-to-get-together-when-we-get-home-and-be-Jewish-together
talk. Rebecca patted me on the back and wished me luck with our
tour guide. Then everyone was gone. I went to a hotel room in Tel
Aviv with only my suitcase and Omer's phone number.

I booked myself nightly—in hopes that for at least one night
I wouldn't be staying there—at the Mugraby hostel. It was forty
dollars a night for a potty-less room, no heat, and a bed with a
sleazy-looking leopard-print comforter. I primped and I preened.
I tweezed and shaved. I prettied myself up as well as I could. It
would all happen so soon—the unfucked would be refucked. I
went to bed.

In the morning, I called Omer from a pay phone. Omer said he
was still feeling too sick, but I think I might have heard a basketball game going on in the background. He said to call him later.
So then I went on a hummus and white bread binge. I knew I was
poisoning my orgasm, but at that moment, I didn't care.

I refused to feel sorry for myself, so I went for some retail therapy. Eric was right; it did divert sexual energy for a while, but not
long enough. And mind you, all this time, I'm calling Omer and

he's still mumbling nonsense through high-fevered pain. Or so he said.

So I continued my orgasmic ancestry search. I thought of Momo Lifshitz, the organizer of the trip. He seemed knowledgeable about loving; plus, he told all the Birthright participants that if we were in need, we could reach him anytime on his cell phone. So I called him and asked him for an orgasm interview.

"It's Shabbat!" he said. Momo could put on a good angry. "Don't you have any respect?"

"Sorry," I said, but he didn't hear me; the phone clicked off before I could put another coin in the slot. I went and sat on my leopard comforter, and then I banged my head on the pillow. I was going to cry, I wanted to cry, I couldn't cry. I needed Rori to cry.

My potential orgasm collaborator was failing me!

The next day I met with a sexologist named Orit Armond. One of the Israeli soldiers had told me about her. We had to meet in her car in the pouring rain because she was running late to give a dildo presentation at a bachelorette party. The bachelorette didn't want me to come along. We had about five minutes together. She talked about masturbation as it applied to Jews. "Jewish law says women should masturbate," she said. "It doesn't say she shouldn't, so she should!"

But Eric's toys wouldn't even have helped; this yearning was much deeper than any plastic could have filled up. I couldn't stop shaking my head back and forth in disbelief at my idiocy. I should have been home in New York by then, fantasizing about what would have happened if I'd stayed in Tel Aviv.

Orit told me sex with your husband is a mitzvah, a commandment, and if people in the United States understood that, they'd preserve more marriages. "In America they do it once a year," she said. "Not enough." Then I remembered something Rabbi Levine had said. He said that the one snag in the whole Jews-are-open-and-orgasmic thing is that it's all meant to happen between two people with wedding bands. "Every classical Jewish text will teach and preach that sex belongs in marriage," the rabbi had said. "Outside is frowned upon. But inside marriage, sky's the limit! It's wonderful." He even said anal was cool as long as you said your vows first.

My orgasmic roots were drying up by the hour. I guess the desert can dry up just about anything.

The final day, I let Omer go. I didn't call. He didn't call. I was a cow from the hummus by that point anyway, which made it all the more odd when my vulva ran away from me; the ring slipped off my pudgy finger and rolled down Ben Yehuda, a wide, busy street. I ran to pick it up. I looked up to the sky. Spiritual gonorrhea—I had a bad case.

I packed up that evening. My plane was early the next morning. I went to Mike's Place, an expat bar next door to the U.S. embassy. I started talking to a Canadian expat named Leah. I told her about my un-affair. She said I was better off anyway; she'd been with a lot of Israeli guys and their idea of "better" was always faster and harder. "I tell them, 'Slowly, slowly, my friend,'" she said, "but they don't listen. They do what they see in the movies. Bam bam bam."

She said that in Hebrew, all nouns are either feminine or masculine and the clitoris, somehow, is referred to as male. "He asked me where *he* was," she said, speaking about a lover searching for her clit. "How can you get the right loving when they think she's a he?"

I think she was just trying to make me feel better. I felt a little better—at least I was returning to a country where my anatomy, like me, could be female.

On the airplane, there was a big Hasidic Israeli man to the right of me. I only asked that I not get a cougher. Of course, I got a cougher. He coughed through his wiry beard, putting out all remnants of twitter I had left between my legs.

Maybe it was better this way; I didn't have to hurt this way. If only I could have talked to Fiona, I would have told her to tell me that everything was going to be okay.

There was a pile of muffins in the plane's galley. I took one and brought it to my seat. I offered the cougher the baked good because I felt guilty. I loathed his phlegm so vehemently that I began to loathe him. I didn't even know him. That wasn't fair.

"Want a muffin?" I asked.

"Why did you take the muffin if you didn't want the muffin?" he asked.

"I thought you might want it," I said. "I was being considerate."

"You weren't hungry and you take a muffin?" he said. "Why did you take the muffin?"

"I was being nice," I said. If I had hackles, they would have been raised.

"If I want to eat a muffin," he said, "I know how to get my own muffin."

I shoved the plastic-covered baked good in the pocket of the seat in front of me.

I exhaled.

Profound. This cougher was deep.

I'M FUCKING HAPPY, DAMN IT!

I stared closely at my follicles, my barren leg follicles. Little black dots. I watched them for a couple days. They don't stay barren for long. The little proteins peeked their black tips above my hide, mocking me for having preemptively chopped them down in my hopes for man company. Little bastardly reminders. Little scornful things.

I contemplated calling Omer overseas to see if he had gotten better, but I'd put myself out enough. I should get an Oscar for my role as desperate girl. I'd be typecast for good if those four days were filmed.

I decided that I should at the least just make sure he hadn't died.

So I Googled him. If he had died, he hadn't done it in English because no Omer obituaries popped up. There was a chance his obituary was written in Hebrew, but at this very moment he was probably entranced by a basketball game, hypnotized by balls swishing through hoops. Balls and hoops . . . balls through hoops . . . balls penetrate hoops . . .

And you know what happened to the poor Collector in the basement? Ursula told me that while I was away, some doctor put our hoarder on pills—and they worked. The Collector's piles were at a standstill. His hoards were stagnating. Stagnation—it almost felt worse than steady baggage accumulation because there was nothing for his mound to do but to go rotten. The junk all turning into one big molten thing.

Fiona, on the other hand, was done stagnating. She finally finished her contract with the show and would be visiting in a week, before she took off to India to find some more pieces of herself. She assured me that Omer wasn't meant to be; the signs were clear, she said. Vomiting was always a pretty clear sign.

Then the inevitable Rori visit happened. I felt my leg hairs graze against my jeans as I settled into her sofa. I told her the whole Omer debacle.

I looked at that Van Gogh print, my eyes swishing along wildly with the brush strokes. Seriously, that was a bad choice for a psychotherapist's office.

"How did you feel about not seeing Omer again?"

"Fine," I said. "It wasn't Omer's fault. He was sick. How could I be mad? It wasn't meant to be, at least it seemed that way."

"Whom are you giving authority to?" she asked. "Whom are you giving rights to, to assign meaning to your life?"

That was a good question because I didn't believe in God. I believed in free will and in a world where ants were indiscriminately squished, yet I'd been writing letters to W. Wall and humping God for the past two weeks . . .

"Aren't you upset that it didn't work out?" she prodded.

"No," I said. "It turned out for the best. I feel like myself now. I've got great dopamine levels. I'm one of those bounce-back people. I bounce right back. I'm happy."

I'M FUCKING HAPPY, DAMN IT!

I gave her a fat smile, teeth-baring and all. "See?"

She said it wasn't all about dopamine levels, though I should take credit for my coping mechanisms. She said I'd developed great ones.

"Thank you," I said. I kept my mechanisms well-oiled and greased. They were constantly in gear. Churning. I could cope. I'm a gold-medal coper.

Then she told me to let my mechanisms rest, put down the need for constant happiness, and feel all the feelings that were coursing through me. She said because my mechanisms were so topnotch, I don't allow myself to feel negative emotions. Sadness, unhappiness, anger—they were coming out in other ways, she said. "It feeds your anxiety, your fear of death," she said. "Those are feelings you've become comfortable with."

"I don't want to be angry," I said. "Isn't the point to be happy? I just want to be happy and feel my sex."

"Anger and turn-on are only a few notches away," she said. "If you don't allow yourself to feel one, you won't fully feel the other."

I wrote her my monthly check with my mechanisms on full alert. I smiled all the way outside. It was a brilliant day. The clouds were gray; a truck huffed exhaust in my face; my hands were going numb from the cold; and a man gave me a flat tire, stepping on the heel of my shoe, as I got into the subway. I beamed at it all. It's a fucking brilliant day, damn it! Just fucking genius.

DON'T STOP. DON'T, STOP.

I had a friend who felt bad about the Omer fiasco. He felt I shouldn't have given up on the Chosen People so quickly, so he signed me up for JDate, an Internet dating site for Jews. So I put up a profile to appease him and maybe a little bit to show myself that I could date men on the same continent. Plus, Atman had me thinking about how everyone needs someone else, even though he's chosen to go through the havoc of life alone.

"You're a part of something more, another person," he'd said. "We need friends, an intimate, a soul mate, know what I mean?"

"But why?" I asked.

"Why?" he said. "Otherwise you pick up self. Be with self. To be with self you need a heck of very long exercises by the way. With self, you need a heck of guts."

I had guts—I might even have a heck of guts—but I had to do something. This was a quest, after all, and I'd been learning that quests never really end. I'd managed to get having an orgasm by myself out of the way, but I still felt like I wanted something more and that something more wasn't only The Gasm's answer to the MEANING OF ORGASM, which still loomed.

It wasn't long before a guy contacted me on JDate. He was hot, almost too symmetrical for my taste. I called Leigh over to my computer, to show her what I'd fetched. She got excited, but then started warning me about dating stuff again. I was glad she was giving me the memos I'd missed. She said hot guys and guys with money could date anyone they wanted. Be strategic. Write sparingly and don't seem too available.

But unfortunately I was quick to the trigger. I'd already written him back.

I broke the rules, it seemed, but he agreed to a drink anyway. We went out and had fun. There were too many glasses of wine involved, which caused cracks in my senses. We kissed in the street. He had a weird little smack on the tail end of his smooches. But he could be trained to retract his tongue in silence, I thought.

I told Leigh about it. She said I was good at dating. She said she thought I could even perfect my skills and become a food whore, going out with men to get free meals. She said men owed us meals and small extravagances because of the eternity in which there had been salary discrepancy between the genders. She used her own methods for achieving gender equality.

I actually got excited about this guy, though, and not just for the meals. I waited for our next date, which we planned for a couple days away, with a little extra spring in my strut. Maybe Omer was just a good primer.

We had dinner, and when we got outside it was raining. I invited him to my house. I'll blame it on Clitty Rose: she was yelping for attention. We were in my room, and I couldn't relax as we made out. He was one of those who thought my breasts were twist-off caps. I thought of Eric and how he'd eased me through it, allowing me to be in control. This felt uncontrollable; this make-out was going somewhere.

"Had many serious girlfriends?" I asked as he nipped my neck. "How has JDate worked out for you? Used the service long?"

I couldn't shut up. Each new question was worse than the one before it. It'd been a while, but apparently I was still very good at subverting a process. I created my distance. In a queen-size bed, I'd managed to make the illusion of us being on separate continents.

He said it was getting late before he even gazed at the green glowing numbers on my digital clock. As he walked down the stairs, the steps groaning beneath him, I felt like my life was on replay. It was the same brown-haired, brown-eyed, medium-built guy going down the stairs over and over again. I didn't know which button to press to make him stop, to make me invite him to stay.

He was too hot anyway.

Find one of your own kind, I thought.

DON'T STOP. DON'T, STOP.

THE SEVEN-YEAR-OLD

Fiona arrived later the next evening. She came in from her final show in Washington D.C. I'd been spending copious amounts of time feeling sorry for myself and trying to hold it together. But when I saw Fiona, my coping mechanisms fell apart. Fucking mechanisms, they aren't built to last.

Fiona stroked my hair as I made a pool of tears in her clavicle. I felt messy. I was hoping it was the kind of mess that was on the way to being a bit more orderly, like the disaster that ensues when you begin sorting out an overly packed closet.

It's a bodily function—only a sensation—yet somehow this orgasm business is attached so strongly to an emotion. This connection has made one very difficult to explore without the other. Love and Orgasm. Logasm. Orgove.

"I'm ne . . . ne . . . ne . . ." I said, my tears preventing an even flow of words, "ne . . . ne . . . ver going to get it right."

I was thinking of men. I seemed to have my man magnet turned the wrong direction; it was repelling these creatures.

All of them, lemminglike, walking in the anti-direction of me.

My father told me that I was one of those types, like him, who would just *know* when I found the right one. I was picky, he told me. But really, how do you know when what you want is in front of you? The only one who had felt right in twenty-six years was Evan, and he only seemed right after we stopped speaking. And I was eighteen.

"You never know for sure," Fiona said. "You just have to dive in and ride the wave."

What if "the one" wasn't what I thought he'd be? I was scared to even attempt finding someone because what if I discovered love wasn't what I thought, wasn't everything I'd expected it to be? Honestly, kind of like the disappointment my first orgasm was.

"Obviously, I got it wrong once already," Fiona continued, "but Mara, relationships are beaaaaautiful things."

She pronounced "beautiful" like she tended to sometimes, extending all the syllables, stretching it out so it could encompass everything. A "beautiful" said like that, like it could float into orbit, made me want to dig my heels in.

"But once you're there," I said, "you're kind of stuck. Where do you go from there? You lose yourself. You end up in a box or in a cul-de-sac."

I took her to my window and told her to look down at The Collector's piles below. "That's stagnation," I said. "That's stuck."

"Stagnation, stuck, losing?" she questioned. "You don't lose yourself. You get to see a whole new side of yourself. Another person brings it out in you. You just have to open up."

"But how do I open up?" I asked her.

"You don't have to try," she said. "I can see you opening up right now."

And I wondered how she'd learned all this stuff. I always thought she'd never been alone long enough to learn about herself.

THE SEVEN-YEAR-OLD

"I feel like the only thing I've figured out in the last five months is that I'm more screwed up than I thought," I said. "I can't make anything work. What if I want to get married someday?"

She held my cheeks and looked at me cockeyed. "You want to get married?" she asked.

"Did I just say that?" I said.

I told her our society's demons had momentarily possessed me. I was speaking in tongues.

Then Fiona told me not to worry about the acne. Worry about being beautiful on the inside, she said.

"I didn't say anything about my acne," I said.

In the morning, Fiona and I followed our tradition. We sat on a stoop, bundled up in sweatpants and down jackets, sipping drip coffee.

That's when I had an existential crisis. You never know when these are going to happen.

Two little boys, I'd say about seven years old, came up to us. One came especially close. He stared at me. He looked carefully at my face, then down to my feet. An older woman, maybe his mom, was further behind. He kept staring.

"Hi," Fiona said. He didn't bat an eyelash in her direction. He was looking intently at me.

Did he have one of those behavioral things—ADHD or Asperger's?

He finally opened his mouth, and with it came the crisis.

"Are you a kid or an adult?" he asked me. He said it with a kind of snotty tone, like it was my fault he didn't know, that I should be more upfront with what I am.

I looked at Fiona for input. She shrugged her shoulders. I furrowed my brow.

"I don't know," I said. "What am I?"

"How old are you?" he asked, jumping up and down.

His mother arrived. "Don't ask ladies their ages, sweetie," she said. "It's not polite."

I told her it was fine. I was desperate for the answer. I needed the answer. He had the answer. How did a little kid have the answer?

"I'm twenty-six," I said. "Kid or adult?"

"You're an adult," he shouted. "Did you like college?"

"Wait, I'm an adult?" I said. "Are you sure?"

His mother took his hand and pulled him away. "I'm so sorry," she said. "Sorry to interrupt you, ladies."

"No," I said. "No, wait, I have more questions! What's the cut-off age?"

He was already up the street, jumping cracks in the pavement.

THE SEVEN-YEAR-OLD

MY SENSITIVE HEART OF STONE

I wanted to call my mom to see if she already knew that I was an adult and badger her about why she hadn't let me in on it yet. But I didn't. Instead I feared death for a while. Then I procrastinated from fearing death by hunting JDate profiles. I wanted to try someone different—maybe a little bit of a freak, but not a sick bastard. My sensitive heart of stone was having trouble opening up to the straightforward hot ones. I found a guy, Hank, who looked interesting and not too symmetrical. Not asymmetrical, exactly, but just enough off-kilter. On my level. We were equally mediocre.

Physical mediocrity is a worthy quality to be born with. The not-too-hot people develop character—we *have* to. A normal gal like me can't get by on only winks.

But I digress.

Hank and I met a couple days later, over a glass of wine. When I first entered the bar, I spotted him with his ear to his water glass. He said he was listening to the room's cacophony through his glass's hollow. He said each glass transforms noise into its own distinctive whirring-type music. "I'm a sound technician," he said, as if that would somehow normalize his actions. When he spoke, he peered over the top of his glasses with big gray orbs. He had a rotund belly that I hadn't quite prepared for; it was those neck-up Internet profile pics. His fuzzy light brown beard framed his round cheeks, seeming to fasten his jowls into place. A hedge of hair was overgrown, obscuring his lips. I'd never dated a guy with so much facial hair before, and I felt it was potential false advertising. What if he was chinless under all that scruff?

He said men must be intimidated by my book topic and then quickly added that his penis was so big it'd been mistaken for a prosthetic leg before.

My face was locked up in laugh-position for so long that by the time we parted, my cheeks were cramping. But Clitty Rose, that bitch, never said anything. And right then, I knew I couldn't kiss him, but he didn't try anyway.

STRAP-ON-VILLE

I met up with Zola that week. Zola had just returned from Dubai with a client. When he was temporarily outsourced, he wanted his orgasm outsourced with him. He put her up in five-star hotels while he did business for a few weeks. She said it was easy; she just butt-fucked him with a strap-on a few times and did some eye-gazing.

I couldn't get that image out of my head—Zola wearing a strap-on. She made it sound so simple, like she'd been asked to go pick up his dry cleaning or something.

I told her about my Hank experience. I felt a conundrum brewing. I said that his personality was great, but arousal wasn't stirring. I said he wasn't perfect, it wasn't love at first sight or anything, not what I thought romantic "like" or "love" could start out looking like, but for some reason, I didn't want to give up on it yet.

"I hate that fairy-tale bullshit!" she said. She pulled her hair down at the tips and looked upward. "It's never perfect. God, the fairy tale fucks everyone up!"

She told me it was a secret, but that even Prince Charming had his defects: he had halitosis, a propensity to drone on about irrelevant shit, and a chronic case of early ejaculation.

"They just don't tell you that part," she said, "because not as many people would go see the movie." She told me the princess had a gag order; she was only allowed to talk about those issues with her therapist.

"Have you tried on a strap-on before?" she asked.

I shook my head.

"You've never tried one on!" she said. "I wish I could give a strap-on to every woman, including my grandmother." She thought it'd help me to relate to men better. She said it would demystify the penis: "A dick is just a dick."

(She also said she'd especially like to give one to every bride. "Someone's got to lose their virginity that night," she said.)

I went to her temple on the Upper East Side a few days later. Pale blue silk with flying geese patterns stitched into it hung from the ceiling. There were two sitting pillows placed on a circular shag carpet, where, during sessions, she'd eye-gaze with clients. She called that, as opposed to buggering someone with a dildo, the most intimate part of her Tantra sessions. A massage bed had bolts of white cloth streaming above it to form a canopy. Plants lined the windowsill, and each wall was painted a different shade of calm.

A leather case and a couple of dildos were on the massage table. "I regret that I don't have more penises," she said. "My friends stole most of my penises."

"That's a big penis," I said. It was pink and the size of my forearm.

"Yeah," she said, "that's Ferris the diamond dealer's cock."

She told me he was a client who loved to go down on himself, but wasn't flexible enough. So she wore a silicon counterpart—

same size—and he used his imagination for the rest. "Yes," she said, "that was very narcissistic, and so very hot!"

She respected all of her clients' quirks and thought of them as no odder than if their desires were dietary concerns and she had to fulfill them as their personal chef.

She said most of the other guys who went down on her strap-on did it for other reasons. "I'm thinking it's mostly a psychological submission thing," she said, nonchalantly. "They associate blow jobs with demeaning themselves. A BDSM thing."

She dug into the leather case and pulled out what looked like a demonic pacifier. It was translucent blue and had tiny spikes all around it. She flipped a switch, it buzzed, and she touched it to her nose. "It's going to make me sneeze," she said. "I swear to God, the best sneezes are vibrator sneezes."

I was tempted to try it but quickly learned it was a butt plug. "It's a little bit addictive," she said. "But at least it's not crack."

She began sneezing. She went to grab a tissue. She counted her sneezes. "Seven sneezes equals an orgasm," she said. "I need two more."

She put the plug to her right nostril; she sneezed twice more to make seven and then put it down. She moaned, caught her breath, and then walked back over to her pile of paraphernalia.

"Okay, strap-on-ville," she said. "There are different kinds of strap-ons. I'm so excited to induct you into strap-on-ness. There's g-string-style. This is more jock strap," she said, holding up a dark red leather harness. "I need to polish this baby up." She bent down so I could put my legs through. She pulled it over my jeans and up to my waist.

"Oh, wait, I'm sorry," she said. "I'm all mommying you. You can put on your own dick. I'm sorry."

She said the first time she put on a cock, she felt unbounded.

"I felt like the world was full of limitless opportunities," she said. "I felt much bigger."

It wasn't about becoming a man—"I love my pussy! I love my pussy!" she assured me—but realizing there was nothing sacred and holy about wielding a cock.

"In such a male-centric culture," she said, "it feels good to take that phallus and say, 'You're not out of my domain.'"

I snapped in my dick, a seven-inch black cock. I leaned my chest forward and swung it back and forth like I was fencing. "Touché!"

"Yeah," Zola said. "Does it feel good? Work it out, man. You could do some damage with that thing!"

I looked in the mirror and checked myself out. Zola took aim at me with a camera.

"Do you think my cock is too big or too small?" I said. It had only been two minutes, and I was already having penis anxiety. I was very aware of where it was, what it was doing. I felt vulnerable about my cock.

"It's really a perfect size for a lot of people," she said, validating my penis. "A little big for an untrained butt, but perfect for girls."

I felt better for a minute, but then I started second-guessing it again when I saw the reflection of myself in the window. "You sure it's a good size?"

When Zola buckles on her strap-ons these days, it's mostly for work. She says that in her work with men, it's very psychologically healing to be a dude and have something in your ass. "Letting another person see your shit," she said, "like literally that's where the shit comes from, 'Oh my god, they can see my shit . . . ahhh,' and all the shame that opens up, and that other person can be so close to something you've protected for so long and not reject you—it feels amazing."

"So you see people's shit?" I asked.

"Every once in a while, yeah," she said. "There are a couple people. Older men who are corporate lawyers tend to be constipated. It's always a bummer if you're wearing a long dick, and you're fucking 'em, and it bumps up against a little brown, and you're like, 'There's shit on the tip of my dick.'"

I took off my black cock and put on Ferris's gigantic dick. It barely fit through the belt's stabilizing ring. "I wouldn't date me if I had a cock this big," I said. I was tilting forward from the mass. "This thing would put any vulva in peril."

I tightened my dick into place. The weight was pulling the belt loose. "When I fuck someone with a strap-on," she said, "it doesn't diminish my femininity, but I feel like such a smart female that I can add onto it."

I sat up on the massage table. My cock folded in between my legs.

"In our culture we have this very artificial thing," Zola said. "The dick is supposed to be like stone, always supposed to be hard, but the cock's not this static unmovable thing. It's beautiful soft, beautiful semi-erect, beautiful hard, beautiful ejaculating. It's cyclic and beautiful in all phases, just like women are."

I spotted a small gouge in the tip. "What's that from?" I asked.

"One of my clients . . ."

"Did he bite it?"

"I asked him to bite it," she said. "Sex can be scary and fucked up. It was so good when he bit it, such a huge release of energy and so nice to approve of him while he went through that."

My cock represented pain to someone. It represented pleasure to others. Fertility to the masses. It was a potent thing.

It was a complicated thing.

She said both sexes had feminine and masculine within them. "I think it's important to try all sides of our natures," she said. "We're not all like soft, feminine, polite, ready to get fucked anytime. We can strap on big dicks and run big companies, and men can be soft, coy, and demure."

She looked at my soft cock. It was lying on the table.

"Oh, my," she said, "you're fondling your dick!"

I looked down. I haven't even noticed. My penis was just so out there, it was hard to ignore.

I couldn't stop touching my cock.

POUNCE-ABLE?

After that visit with Zola, I started waking up on the other side of my bed—waking up by the heater instead of by my side table. Was that a sign? Was I finding my other half—the masculine side of me—or was I just freezing, half-consciously scooting toward warmth?

Around this time, Samantha from the Orgasm People got back in touch with me. She must have sensed the Saber's vibrations. I'd taken out my appliances a few times, letting my index finger go by the wayside.

Samantha said she'd convened with the family and they wanted to offer me a scholarship for their next communication course, which was one week away. All I had to do was buy a plane ticket. I had mixed feelings: Was this merit-based or affirmative action for the orgasm-challenged?

Since this was a communication course, I called them back and asked if I could stay an extra day for some guidance. "I'd like some orgasm tutoring," I said. I wanted to supplement my orgasm knowledge, building onto what I'd already learned. I felt ready for Orgasm Level Two.

"Tell us what you want and we will accommodate you," Samantha said.

Before I left, I saw Hank a few more times.

I began to see how Hank had made it to thirty-three years old without getting hitched. For our second date, he showed up a half hour late to our sushi dinner—he napped beyond his alarm bell—but he made up for his tardiness by telling me about a type of coffee that is brewed from the beans collected from the shit of a small mammal called a civet that eats the coffee berries. "It takes out some of the acidity," he said of the already-been-digested beans. "A smooth blend!" He said he'd be happy to make me a cup. Then he went on to tell me that he wanted to have children, but said it by using the word "spawn" and continued the thought with, "I want to spray someone's eggs with my sperm." Somehow I found it endearing how he walked the line between gross and funny, obscene and interesting. It seemed as if he'd missed a few years' worth of memos himself.

We still hadn't kissed by our sixth date, which was crazy and also the last date before I was going back to Orgasm Camp. He met me in my neighborhood. We grabbed coffees and then settled in my room to talk. We sat on my bed for about an hour, the coffee almost gone and the sun setting, reflecting a pinkish gold off the Brooklyn buildings. Time was running out and he hadn't even touched me yet.

"Are you going to kiss me or am I going to have to do it?" I asked.

"I like to wait until it's overly awkward before I kiss someone," he said.

He didn't make any kissing noise at all. I could retrain him to make at least a little suction sound. And he didn't keep kissing me.

POUNCE-ABLE?

He relaxed and began looking out the window again. Why wasn't he trying to pounce on me like other men? I didn't like it when men pounced, but at the same time, I wanted to be pounce-worthy. Am I not pounce-able? Maybe he just had more control. Maybe he was just more mature. He was obviously more mature than I was; I bit him, blew raspberries on his arm, and accidentally drooled on his hand.

He took it okay.

When it was time for him to leave, I was concerned about walking him out. I didn't want to hear those groaning stairs again. But I didn't have to because as he went down the steps, he tripped. He chuckled sheepishly, overriding the stairs' squeaky pitch.

I still questioned our compatibility—I wanted to want him—but I'd have to figure it out when I got back from Orgasm Camp. I'd invited Zola to come along, and she had agreed to accompany me to Pussy Willow Ranch.

As I was about to take off, Fiona was making final preparations for India. She called me in a freak-out. She was nervous about going to a new place alone. Our roles were reversed; I felt as comfortable traveling alone in foreign countries as she was in the coital embrace. Oddly, the counsel I gave her for her trip closely resembled the advice she often gave me about relationships. "Just ride the wave," I said. "Be open to what happens. No expectations. Trust yourself."

IT'S A FRIENDLY THING TO DO

It was 2:03 p.m. PWCT (Pussy Willow Creek Time). I waited in the cottage. Collin was three minutes late. If they could be wrung out, my palms felt clammy enough that they'd fill a tumbler. Charlotte agreed to sit with me while it happened. Eloisa and Neil were there too; he was in a blue terrycloth bathrobe and had just finished off a plate of pancakes. He'd slathered butter on them from the rim inward. "I'm an edge butterer," he said. "Pleasure first. None of that middle saving-the-best-for-last bullshit." He said my cheeks were flushed; it was a sign of turn-on.

"I'm nervous," I said. Neil snapped off pink quince blossoms from a branch sitting in a vase. "Stop acting naïve," he said. "You can't be naïve anymore. Stop it!" I was about to defend myself when I saw Collin through the window; he was approaching with a box of rubber gloves in one hand and a gigantic tube of lube in the other. Collin's a DO-er. Anyone can be, but I guess he's a professional of the Deliberate Orgasm. For the past twelve years, he's DONE women one to eight times a day. That means that since I was a freshman in high school, his index finger has been responsible for anywhere between 4,380 to 35,040 orgasms. If orgasms are stars, he's accountable for a small fraction of a galaxy. My brows bunched so tightly that I felt my ears pull toward my nose. "Now get in there and have fun!" Neil ordered. "Fun!"

I tipped my head against Eloisa's shoulder, trying to steal some of her mojo, as if it could be transferred through skin, before going inside the bedroom.

Zola had left early that morning to catch a flight from San Francisco; we'd spent the past two days attending the communication course with the Orgasm People.

On the first night, I noticed that not much had changed since I had been there three months before; I believe Caleb even had on the same sweater. There was still lots of laughing. Laughter must be the tangible form of excess orgasm; it lay like a fog in their living room. They laughed at everything—uninhibited throw-their-head-back-until-I-can-see-clearly-into-their-nostrils kind of laughter—especially when I didn't get the joke. Like when I asked why they had given me a scholarship.

"Is it because I'm a good student, or did you think I desperately needed help?"

"Neither," Samantha said.

"Aww," I said. "It's because you guys like me."

Neil cleaned the underside of his fingernails with his pocket-knife and then got up to leave the room. "I can't go saying that," he said. "Then you'll think I want to fuck you."

I had a good two and a half minutes to check them all out; the Orgasm People have clean nostrils.

Again, the food was unbelievable. The Pussy Willow Creek Ranch deserves to be rated by the Michelin Guide. The cuisine looks no better than a diner's, but it hits the spot like a Thanksgiving feast would after a famine—and they aren't afraid of butter, fat, or sugars (as became particularly apparent as I watched them prepare duck confit, cramming roasted duck legs into mason jars already filled to the rim with yellow gelatinous lipids). They seemed to eat all day but kept their trim figures. Neil said knowing their orgasm put them into a state of just being. "They don't have to insulate themselves from anything," he said, referring to the women in the family. "Others eat and get fat; it's a way of insulating from whatever they are trying to hide from."

That first evening, Zola moaned higher than her usual food-mastication register as we ate dinner. I also made love to the food as I had the time before, but then I spotted Collin, and specifically his pointer finger, at the southwest curve of the table, spooning beef barley stew into his mouth. That finger . . . the finger . . . the finger . . .

I wanted to know, I wanted to experience whatever it was that made them all stick around in the woods and live in a community with orgasm as their everything—sustenance, conversation, livelihood, and bond. It almost seemed wrong—where's Murphy's Law in their world?—to live a life with so much pleasure; it seemed like something would have to go bad. I wondered, if I went under the finger, would I cancel my flight home and become a member of the Orgasm People's community? I didn't know how to ask to experiment—was it inappropriate?—so I mitigated what might have been perceived as my personal interest by couching my question in pure journalistic curiosity.

"Do the Orgasm People ever DO their students?"

I didn't get an answer, but I did get another chance to check out their nasal hygiene.

The point of the course that Zola and I took was to learn how to communicate with attention and intention. To have intention, you have to know first what you want to communicate. The first homework assignment was to put our intention, without words, on something or someone during our lunch break and observe the reactions. We went on a walk and saw their swine, Mountain Girl and Betty, along with thirteen newborn piglets. Collin pointed them out, and as he did, I focused intently on the back of his neck and squinted while chanting *DO me, DO me, DO me* in my head. He didn't turn around until some mud had flung off the backside of his boots as he slopped through the pig goop. He said sorry. When he said sorry, he *did* smile . . . so maybe half the message reached?

It wasn't anything romantic. Collin didn't do to me what Omer had done—my crotch wasn't ready to hijack all rationale in pursuit of touch—but for the Orgasm People, DOing was a friendly activity anyway. If they sold T-shirts, they'd read, "It's a friendly thing to DO."

We took the course with five other people, three of whom were men from the OP's extended community. They lived with two other OP women in San Francisco. Neil seemed particularly concerned that each woman in his community was getting DONE well. Being DONE well, and consistently, equated to well-being and happiness. He believed that if every woman was DONE on a regular basis, the pharmaceutical industry would lose a large portion of their dependable and depressed female client base.

"How is DOing?" Neil asked, directing his question toward a tall svelte man during one of our breaks. "I thought you'd have some questions by now."

The man replied that he often got spaced out while he was DOing. "Does that mean that she's spaced out?"

They said if all attention were focused on the other person, with enough practice, the two people would share the same feelings.

"Of course that means she's spaced out," Neil said. "Flick her clit!"

Then he laughed. They all laughed. And at that moment, my mother and father became bona fide sexual conservatives in my mind.

The course itself was a bit boring for me, but I didn't say that aloud because they have this rule that says that if you're bored, it means you're boring, because all your attention is on yourself. I didn't want them to think I was boring. The whole day we sat face to face repeating the same sentences—*Do fish swim. Do fish swim. Do fish swim.*—over and over again in monotone, with no vias, which meant no facial movements, not even blinking. My eyes were dry, and this time, it wasn't because I was turned on.

So when the course was over and Zola packed up and prepared to leave early in the morning with the other students, I finally had my chance to make something orgasmic happen. The guys hopped in the car, while she was left standing in the foyer. "I'm going to have to work on that intention thing a little more," she said, pointing to the baggage the boys did not help her with. "Or shit, I'm just going to have to train them." She neared the car and turned red, not embarrassed, her face reflecting the trunk's brake lights as she waved them back outside to help her load her suitcase. As she zoomed up the driveway, having got what she wanted, I went down to the brown house for breakfast.

Everyone retrieved his or her own meal—granola, yogurt, bacon, eggs, oatmeal, and coffee. They milled around in their bathrobes for a while, soaking in the sun, which filtered through the pines outside, lackadaisically dappling the front living room. I figured I'd given them every sign possible, except saying it aloud, that I wanted to be DONE. They were always intuitive, but this time they were letting me down.

IT'S A FRIENDLY THING TO DO

They let me dawdle aimlessly. I scooted around, bonking back and forth between rooms, with no goal in mind, like a pinball operated by a blind man. Julia and Kate were making a new thirty-gallon batch of beer. I hovered over them and whined about how much I had to do when I got home. Julia saw my ant tattoo and pointed. "At least you're not an ant," she said, always seeing the bright side. "You won't get squished under someone's shoe."

I moved on.

While Collin and Caleb worked on remodeling the kitchen, Dolly was cooking something. I guessed on an average day, they were just average people; they didn't strip off all their scoop-neck sweaters, which acted as cleavage embroidery, and perform orgies in the garden. There was a small part of me that had entertained that suspicion.

Finally, Rena asked me if I wanted to go on a walk. She wanted to go to Pussy Willow Creek to see if the watercress had grown enough to transform the floating stems into a side dish. Green sprigs popped up under our feet. Her bright blue eyes matched her cable-knit sweater. As we strolled around the blocks of ice, still unmelted from the extraordinary winter freeze they'd had, I kept trying to tell her that I wanted to be DONE, but every time I opened my mouth, my heart jumped and the words melted into my lungs.

She finally spoke, breaking the outdoor symphony of cracking twigs and growling winds.

"You can make happen what you want to happen," she said as our feet sunk into the mulch-laden ground. "Anything can happen."

We passed a nanny goat named Dolce; Rena was close to her. She squeezed her tits every fall to make goat-milk lattes.

"How does one go about getting DONE?" I finally asked. "Or getting a DO date. Or . . ."

"What do *you* want?" she said, smiling. "Just say what *you* want."

"I want one," I said.

She said all I had to do was ask. "We all had the feeling already anyway," she said.

As we neared the house, Julia and Kate, busy brewing, smiled like they knew something was going on. Rena and I entered the front door; somehow, seeing the twelve pairs of boots lined up by the foyer reminded me I was in a sex commune. This place was so weird, but so special. It was like they exploited everything fundamentally human—eating, fucking, feeling, connecting—and would take nothing less than the real. It made so much sense; they lived like humans used to, in tribes, where their foremost preoccupation was taking care of one another. This form of living occurred before we all got caged up in apartments and our foremost preoccupation became making money so that we then could afford Internet dating accounts to meet one another in cyberspace and do what people had originally done naturally.

They kept their day pretty flexible because the urge for a DO could happen spontaneously and almost always took priority. Collin was in the kitchen, making a burrito, when I asked him. Dolly watched me stutter and transform my voice, decibels higher, until it resembled those girls in high school, whom I so hated, when they drew the boys' attention by screeching for help when a bee came close.

"Yes," he answered with a grin. He had to drop the burrito down his throat first. He said he'd meet me at the cottage at two p.m. PWCT.

Collin entered just as I'd brushed my head against Eloisa's shoulder. He followed me into the bedroom, closely accompanied by Charlotte, who, like a Lamaze coach during a birth, would act as my guide and support during my first DO session.

IT'S A FRIENDLY THING TO DO

Charlotte and Collin decided that my first DO date should go for five minutes. (A DO date, as exemplified during the OIC, could go from seconds to days, supposedly.) Charlotte sat on the left-hand corner of the mattress and watched the clock while Collin concentrated on his strokes.

"I'm going to do a little research of my own," I heard Neil call out, which was quickly punctuated by giggles coming from the other side of the wall.

I took off my pants but kept my shirt on. I pulled it down to hide myself, and then I thought about what Neil had said. Was I just acting naïve? After all, I did desperately desire to do the DO, and now it was finally happening. I let go of my shirt's hemline and let it spring up to my waist. I hopped on the mattress; they nodded approvingly and tucked pillows all around my body. I bent my knees and let them fall open. Collin sat by my side and slipped one leg underneath mine. "That's the standard DO position," said Charlotte.

Collin put on the latex gloves, snapping each finger into place— ten snaps and we were ready to go. Just like our communication exercises had taught us in the previous two days, everything he said was in an even tone; it had no value judgment.

He said my pubic hair looked like a Mohawk. I had a punk rock pussy. He took one hand and placed it underneath my butt; with the other hand he lubed me up and then got to stroking.

If I didn't know what he was looking at, I would have thought he was working furiously on a Sudoku puzzle. He was concentrated and straight-faced.

"There's a firmness in your shaft," he said.

"Deep breaths," said Charlotte. "Let your butt sink into the bed."

As they commented on each thing that happened in my body, they helped me stay focused on my crotchular area instead of where my mind seemed to want to go, which was a phrase that seemed to come up again and again on this journey: *What the fuck am I doing?*

"I'm going to lighten those strokes," he said, "take you on a peak."

"Your face is getting flushed," said Charlotte.

"Your lips are engorging," he said.

Charlotte's face was serene. She watched Collin work. The longer we went, the more I wanted it to go on. I wondered if she could move the clock back. It's not so bad to have someone rub your clit, emotion-free, but I did miss the emotion. I looked at Collin's face, and it wasn't someone I wanted to kiss. I briefly thought of Hank.

Maybe love wasn't what I thought, but maybe I could expand the idea of love, like the OP did orgasm, so I could fit more possibilities inside. I wondered how Hank would feel about the DO.

"You're engorged now," Collin said. "About an inch thick. There's a popping sensation when your clit goes through my fingers."

He moved his finger slightly back and forth; the movement was so subtle it wasn't even visible from my vantage point. "Boink," he said. "Right there. Feel it?"

And I felt a little nerve in my leg spasm. My punk rock pussy tightened like it was trying to lip-sync. For the OP, orgasm isn't necessarily achieved by going over the edge but rather by exploiting and prolonging the height of sensation, which occurs on the edge of the edge. I was riding the edge.

"Boink," he said. "Right there."

"Oh," said Charlotte. "She liked that. That felt good."

"I'm getting repositioned under your hood," Collin said. "Oh, you've got a nice mauve tone there now. Now it's turning kind of watermelon."

Charlotte motioned to the clock. It was time for Collin to finish up.

"I'm taking you down now," he said, making longer and heavier strokes. "That's a good landing."

I felt like I'd steamed in a sauna for a half hour. My body was relaxed, but my clit felt like a maraca in mid-shake—tons of little beans were bouncing around in there.

Collin took a dew towel and pressed it on my pubis (or as I had learned in Israel, my FUPA).

I grinned. I saw the expression reflected back to me in their own faces.

I stuck out my hand. I guess that wasn't customary after a DO because I got a very reluctant, yet agreeable, high-five from each of them.

"Now what do I do?" I asked Charlotte, lying slumped in my little nest of pillows.

"Whatever you want," she said. "Appreciate the good feeling in your body."

I felt good—tingles in my chest and some little stems of sensation rooting their way from my groin toward my knees.

"That's a part of our daily life," said Charlotte. "I feel the desire build and then I have a DO date. Anytime I want, I get it."

"And from a man's perspective," said Collin, "when a woman wants one, I can feel it. It's a sensation. I feel Rena right now."

Collin and Charlotte left me to swab up the rest of the excess lube, which had turned my little Mohawk into more of a Jheri curl, and pull up my pants. When I was finished, I went down to the brown house, where everyone meandered around, ready to pounce and ask how my first DO date went.

I told Rena it was great.

"Why don't you ask for another?"

I told her I was leaving that night, in just a few hours.

"It's still possible," she said. "Anything is possible. You just have to ask for it."

Easy enough. I tapped Collin on the shoulder. "Five o'clock?" I said with raised eyebrows. He happily obliged.

These women had it made; they could tap any of the guys on the back at any moment and get their clits rubbed.

"Five minutes, again?" asked Charlotte when we were back in the cottage.

"Six," I said, as Collin snapped his gloves on.

After the second DO date, I was left alone again. I had some slices of cheddar cheese; it was so good I thought it must have been homemade. I looked on the front: Trader Joe's. I guess everything just tastes richer with orgasm around it.

I had to pack up; Eloisa and Charlotte were driving me to the airport. Maybe the reason I felt so much more comfortable with them than with OneTaste—since they did, after all, engage in similar activities—was that I could leave. The OP, like most men I tended to go for, didn't live in my city. It was safe to enjoy them when they were a long flight away because, let's face it, I couldn't really imagine myself living with them. I mean, a part of me could imagine me constantly pulling off my pants—hedonistic, like having every bite be one saturated with butter. But still, spending all day rubbing the clit? I thought it would hardly satisfy my ambitions. Think of my headstone:

RIP: SHE HAD GOOD ORGASMS.

I didn't want to be remembered that way; there was more to accomplish. Plus, there were parts of life at the Orgasm People's ranch that didn't work for me. Primarily, I don't like sharing.

Once my stuff was packed, I made my rounds, saying bye to each of them. No one said much, but their hugs did. They expressed themselves through bodily contact. They soaked me up while squeezing so tight that they sunk into me, so melded that if I had a stink, it would surely become their own. One more crush and then they let go, leaving me with something I didn't have before. Neil stood near the kitchen, looking out the window. He was collecting whatever it was he amassed under his fingernails with his pocketknife again. Maybe the practice was about being considerate; he wanted to be sure his DOing finger was constantly groomed.

"Thanks for having me here," I said.

"Thanks for coming," he said as he looked away, off toward Pussy Willow Creek.

The car was waiting, revved in the driveway.

"Maybe seven minutes next time," I said to Collin, moving toward the door.

"Let's not get too carried away," he said. "Six and a half."

Everyone's nostrils, I'm happy to relate, were still clean.

I hopped in the car; Charlotte hit the gas pedal that would take me back to my world, where Murphy's Law subsisted with those who always expect the worst. I liked that world. I missed it. You never knew if you were going to get squished.

As we finally drove into civilization, where my phone could get reception, I received a text. It was from Hank; he said he was excited to see me.

Charlotte dropped me at the curb. They both got out for one more farewell hug. Eloisa's hair smelled tart and a bit savory. I wheeled my suitcase toward my terminal's entry.

There was orgasm in the hair.

BEARD DANDRUFF

Hank and I dug into warm mushroom salad. The taste was superb mixed in with the creaminess of avocado. I was busy explaining DOing. He laughed at the idea, rolled his eyes backward. He said it sounded wanky, kind of impersonal, too, like farmers beating off their own livestock for artificial insemination. "Too sterile," he said. "I don't jack off my girls like they're swine."

He didn't get it. And truthfully, I probably didn't completely, either. But I was protective of the Orgasm People. I took his disregard as an affront to their orgasmic highness. I didn't tell him I was considering, though maybe I was, taking up DOing as a practice. I could think of worse hobbies.

I had been so looking forward to seeing Hank again—I thought I liked him—but now all I could think about was his beard. Kissing him this time around felt like making out with a moose that'd just dumped its snout into a river—wet and prickly. Little white particles hid in his strands. I picked one away and held it for him to see, my eyebrows raised.

"Beard dandruff," he explained.

I rubbed it off against my jeans, gave a half-ass smile, and forgot to blink for a minute. Even his smell—I didn't think our bodily perfumes mixed well together. That was not an auspicious sign. I'd read it in an article somewhere: olfactory discrimination might foreshadow genetic compatibility. I couldn't help but think in the long term: if I chose to breed, I didn't want to have a pheremonal disaster of a zygote. There were enough obstacles for healthy mitotic growth these days.

"You okay?" he asked, eating a purple potato; it was the color of a person's veins. I remembered Omer's hands. I'd wanted to trace his vessels with my fingertip all the way down to his . . .

"You seem a bit detached," Hank continued. "Kind of disconnected."

A moose with beard dandruff: Acceptable.

A friend with beard dandruff: Acceptable.

A potential lover with beard dandruff: Not acceptable.

A partner, a reflection of the self? As unwilling and unhealthy as that viewpoint was, I saw it that way. He was getting closer and closer to me, impinging on my dandruff-free identity.

I was being hypercritical. I was amassing my list of things not to like. Soon I could distance myself and plead for Rori to help me mourn why it hadn't worked out.

I put my fork down. I lifted my cocktail. We'd ordered fancy sangria. We were celebrating. I was back after a long weekend at Orgasm Camp. We were together again. So many dates—at least seven now—all from an Internet connection. That was something. What a celebration.

I fished around in my glass for an apple chunk.

Hank swung his legs. We were on barstools. There was a widening abyss between us; he had to speak out. "I'm used to being the star in my own story," he said, referring to my book. "I don't know how I feel about taking a supporting role in someone else's." He had a point. Sometimes I didn't even trust myself to be my narrator. And damn it, I grieved over not being omniscient. I wanted to know what everyone else was thinking. Can't have everything, unless you create harmony like the Orgasm People. I'd had a dream since I returned where they were all in a red convertible. Sunglasses on. Arms flailing. Index fingers, like magic wands, pointing toward any roadside object. Just by agreeing on it, they were transforming nouns into verbs at every moment. Anything that they wanted, they changed their joint reality to have it.

Hank asked me if he could be a three-testicled McDonald's cook in the book, to veil his true identity. "I'm private," he said. Honestly, I wouldn't want to date some schmuck who wanted to be in a book. Anyone who liked this kind of scrutiny would be sick (sick like me, I guess). We both agreed on his new identity, so I granted him the title—the three-testied burger flipper—but for all I knew, he could've had the extra testicle. We'd been on numerous dates, but we still hadn't yanked off our clothing yet.

"I'm not used to talking about orgasm in the abstract so much," he said. I think he was hinting. I looked at his belly as he pulled another fungi toward his dandruff. It was like he had half a Pilates ball in there. Overeating, it's a sin in this city, but only when the effects take up residence in the body. But who was I to complain?

We walked toward his apartment. We kissed on a corner while the red-lit hand blinked, telling us not to cross. It wasn't safe. I felt it again, that beard, so feral. He invited me up to his apartment. I saw the sign for the subway. "Later," I said, hugging him all sweet-like, as if I wasn't thinking the things I'd been thinking all night. I rushed down the stairs without looking up. I knew I had boundary issues, but I wasn't sure what kind. When Rori asked me about

BEARD DANDRUFF

boundaries, I could only tell her about the image that popped up in my mind. I thought of a lasso lying on the floor in a circle, and I was standing about three feet outside.

I hadn't had SEX in so long. It'd been almost a year now. (When I told Hank that, he said he was going to call the PPA— Pussy Protection Agency. He said he was a registered foster penis.) I'd traveled too far from the primordial soup bowl.

So I banged myself that night. I'd been lazy that way. My whole orgasmic problem had sprung forth in part because I'd expected someone else to do the work. I thought boyfriends would give it to me so I wouldn't have to excavate it myself. I swirled the Saber around. I was on my bed, with a towel down. The bottle of lube Eric had brought me, still half full, was spilling as I kneaded away. I felt a little guilty about using the vibrator after having just come from a community that ran on fingers only. When I'd talked to Zola about vibrator addiction, she said I shouldn't worry, but she told me when she begins to feel dependent, she implements a two-week vibrator fast. "It's your choice, lady," she said.

Climax wasn't coming easily. I was thinking: This story is coming out all wrong. I'm sexing with the sex people, I'm sexing all by myself, but I'm not sexing with the love people, the people who really give a shit. Something was turned upside down, and it wasn't just the Saber, which was cantering like a prissy pony over my clitty.

I lay there, naked. I smelled the tip of my machinery. Fiona says she's always trying her pussy juices so she can keep up with her cycle changes. I like my pussy now, I do, and I can snuffle up, even enjoy her fragrance—her twinkle—just fine, but I'm not going to put her in my digestive tract. I'm just not; don't expect me to. I like keeping some boundaries intact.

HANK MEETS EARL

I forbade Eric, and every past intimate other, to near my umbilicus region, ever. No navel. It was just a rule I've always enforced. Touching it makes me bilious inside. Eric, apparently, couldn't accept the reality of an off-limits epidermal area, so he'd sought out the advice of a navel specialist and forwarded me her response. He said he wanted to get together soon to explore the repressed emotions pent up in the little knot, which was quite possibly a result of the Western practice of preemptive cord-cutting—that was only one of the specialist's many guesses—and also to conduct routine maintenance on my masturbation form. But it'd have to wait for a bit, he said, because the man who first introduced Betty to sex while using a vibrator, a pivotal moment in her development as a sex philosopher, had just passed away. They were in mourning.

Meanwhile, I desperately wanted to want Hank. I wanted to want him so bad. At the same time, I tried to scare him away. I tried to tell him everything unpleasant about me. I told him I sniffed my pits to get inspired. I told him I stole Shanghai dumplings with my fingers from grocery stores. I told him I liked to wear Groucho glasses with the big nose and fuzzy black mustache to formal affairs. But Hank continued to call me—I can't tell you why. I would have been through with me by now. If I had to wait a month and a half for me to put out, compounded by the prospects of a public unveiling of all my insecurities and bedroom tactics, I'd dump me immediately. Immediately. Actually, if one could dump oneself, I probably would have already chucked my shit to the curb by now. We were seeing each other every other day, though. Something had me coming back. I was surprised each time I found myself there, sitting across from him or lapping up his essence with my mouth. We made an awful saliva compound together. I even asked Ursula what she thought about the matter. You can't live with a bad slobber mixture. It must mean something.

"Stick it out," she said. "Things can change if you give it time."

"Has it ever happened to you?" I asked her.

"No, not really," she said. "But I dated a guy once who never washed his feet."

"And how'd that go?" I asked.

"It was nasty," she said. "We broke up after a few weeks."

"Oh."

I was over at Hank's apartment. "I like my girls dense like I like my banana bread," he said as he squeezed my thigh. I had absolutely nothing to say to that, but I still stayed near. I think he was trying to scare me away too because his home was the concrete expression of repulsion; it was a disaster zone. So many things were stacked on the floor that I needed a shovel to discover if there was carpeting or hardwood below. I swear it wasn't lint on his sofa but a buildup of particulate matter expelled from his facial hair. His laundry pile was so tall it peeked over the top of his incredibly high mattress.

I could clean this place up. It needed a feminine touch, that's all. Wait, what was I thinking?

I called my mom. "I like him, Mom, I think. But I think there's a problem. Maybe we're not physically compatible."

"It drives me crazy," said my mom, not even acknowledging my line of thinking. "Why don't women like nice guys?! You want someone mean? I don't get it. It's stupid. Stupid. Stupid."

"Thanks, Mom," I said.

She was just upset because her biological clock was tick tick ticking for a grandbaby.

Then Hank was back at my place, not even two days later. It was late and we were in my room and I really didn't want him to sleep over. We'd be crossing into the lasso space, my boundary, which I refused to share. I liked waking up by myself, not rocking to the gait of someone else's night twitches. And snoring—I abhor it. I'm a light sleeper. What if he snored? Did he realize it'd be over instantly if he had the slightest problem with his sinuses?

It took imminent separation to kick-start passion because just as I was about to kick him out, we started kissing. This time our make-out finally had an engine. We were pressed so firmly that it felt like his barbs were sinking into my own follicles—impossible to tell which of us had the whiskers. He said we made out like high school kids. I asked what that meant. He said that we kissed forever. I asked, how do adults make out then? He said they don't make out that long.

"That's a shame," I said.

Clothes came off. It was not graceful: reluctantly executed decisions about who unbuckled whom, shimmying and squirming out of our cotton cocoons. I was nervous to see his flesh in the flesh. Nervous about how he'd react to my body, about how I'd react to his belly protrusion. But he was as gentle as the Pillsbury Dough-

HANK MEETS EARL

boy—if not quite so white—and I wanted to poke him to hear his giggle. And I did, and he did. Hank's a ridiculously ticklish man.

He touched me and it didn't feel systematic; at least I didn't feel like livestock. He felt around in my humid excitement and asked if I liked it. I didn't want to tell him. I'd forgotten how normal people interact with vulvas. He was the first amateur clit rubber in quite a long time who was doing so as a method of showing affection. I'd acquired almost an anthropological interest in clitoral stimulation techniques by now.

I knew that I had to stimulate him, too, or at least I felt that was the appropriate thing to do. Maintaining the status quo through quid pro quo genital manipulation, to get Latin about it. Or maybe I just wasn't ready for his undivided attention. So we were facing each other, his hand on my cooter, doing something like figure eights (the OP would freak about his off-the-clit abandon) and me, with my go-go-gadget arm flexibility to get around to his testicular tent.

A dyad! He wasn't a mutant, though don't think I'm not open to that.

He looked different horizontal. I felt a corneal connection. They let me jump in. I was swimming in softness. In tenderness. He wanted to take me in.

Then he jizzed. I'd leaned away so I wouldn't incur splash-back.

His fingers hovered, twittering, in the air.

"More?" he asked me.

What a conscientious guy.

"No, I'm fine," I said.

He looked inspired to supplement my sensations, but he didn't push it. I understood the curiosity; here I am talking about coming all the time like it's my long-lost best friend, and here he is, giving me a chance to hang out with her again, and I decline. But I was ninety-nine percent positive my orgasm was still going to be stingy with new people. I was just pleased we'd managed to take off our pants.

We were both naked. I looked down toward my groin. I'm hairy down there. I asked Hank what he thought of my Mohawk. "Is it all right?"

Instead of answering, he told me about a pubic hair wig called the merkin, which apparently my bush reminded him of. People, especially prostitutes, used to wear them to hide the scars left from various venereal diseases, he said.

He knew the exact wrong thing to say. I kind of loved it.

Then we cuddled.

But then he suddenly looked toward my left armpit with horror. I looked down, terrified at what I might find there. Did I forget to shave? Did I reek? But it's my right pit that usually has the *real* stink. Then I saw what he saw. Guess who was there: Earl the Stuffed Elephant, cradled in my arm. How'd he get there? I was sandwiched between Earl and Hank, holding them both. I got a little flustered.

"That's Earl," I said. He laughed.

It was three-thirty a.m.

"You better get going," I said. "If you want to make it back. Is that okay?"

"I mean, I'd rather stay," he said. "But it's fine, no problem."

It couldn't be only the hairy little number between my legs he was after; his limited access would hardly be worth all this patience.

And he really wasn't at all miffed about getting the pre-dawn boot. And I thought, holy shit, I'm a terrible person. I bet The Collector wouldn't even kick out his hoards of trash into the backyard at this hour.

HANK MEETS EARL

THE PUSSY WHISPERER WOULD LIKE ALL WOMEN TO TASTE HIS CHOCOLATE CAKE

Hank and I weren't monogamous; we hadn't decided titles yet. Well, we hadn't really talked about it. My dating profile was actually still up on the Internet. My subscription had a few more weeks left. Too lazy to take it down? Still curious to see what might pop up?

So I didn't feel guilty when Eric showed up, looking kind of dashing in the yellowish candlelight. We were in my room again. In tiny vials, he'd brought over what he called sex oils. Ylang-ylang, one was called. Exploiting olfaction to aid turn-on. It smelled musky, earthy, almost lewd.

We'd been planning this rendezvous for a while, before Hank and I had taken off our pants. So I didn't feel guilty. This was for my education. Eric was a teacher, remember: a carnal professor.

But he looked more like a sex superhero as he lifted his customary spandex shirt—BODY ARMOR embossed on the breast—over his head. We flopped on the bed. He said we should free-style cuddle—just squirm around to find new ways to fit together. The music was on; he believed in accompaniment. Ambiance. Mood management.

It was so much easier for me to be uninhibited with him than with Hank. Eric's head faced down on my chest, and he used his hands to scrunch my feet. "This one is fun," he said of our newfound position.

We'd just gone out to dinner, Thai food. He still clung to his bedroom and beyond-the-bedroom duality of comportment. Without a bed in his vicinity, he wasn't quite a blind person without a cane but, at the most awkward moments, reminiscent of one.

We caught up. It'd been three months since he'd given me the Saber. He told me about some syrupy crystal hard-ons he'd had (his adjectives). I told him about Hank.

"I'm finally dating someone," I said.

He asked me if Hank had a beer-can cock.

"A lot of women I know love the Jewish beer can," he said.

I asked what that meant.

He said Jewish penises had the reputation for being not so long but fat.

I envisioned Hank with a Budweiser can as a cock, and then quickly shook my head to dispel the vision. I wondered what kind of Jews Eric had been hanging out with.

We walked side by side back to my apartment. He towered over me; his hip pivoted in my curve like a ball bearing in a socket.

We were still on cock talk. He said he thought women had a thing for big penises because there's a magical spot on the cervix—way up in there—that when thumped, gives unique sensations. "Like Christmas lights going on," he said. Betty had told him all about it.

I said I wouldn't mind if Christmas lights accompanied my twinkle, but he was already onto the next thing. He said women told him he had a nice cock. "Is that something that girls learn at girl school?" he asked. "Do they learn to tell guys that they have a perfect cock?"

THE PUSSY WHISPERER WOULD LIKE ALL WOMEN

How do you respond to that without condemning yourself to having lied during some (or all) past penis appraisals?

"Girl school," I said. "Funny." Repeating, as I had learned from parrots, always got you out of answering.

After cuddling, I took two drops of ylang-ylang and started massaging him. He warned me that he'd been taking too many omega-3s and the oils had caused extra hair growth on his ass. "Six a day is too much," he said, cautioning me. He said he had started shaving; he was even contemplating laser hair removal.

Even sacred whores have self-conscious moments. That made me feel oddly triumphant; only a few hours before, I'd cursed at my happy trail while I took a swipe at it with a home waxing kit.

Eric worked out so much that he'd developed the prototype man ass. I didn't think it was just the ylang-ylang essence that had me thinking that. It bubbles up like a perfect bell curve, the apex perpendicular to his spine. In fact, his body might have been a prototype sex body. His mouth was so versatile and Gumby-like that he could fit anything inside. He had my whole tit—they aren't so massive, but still, that was impressive—in his mouth a minute ago. "Spiritual nursing," he'd mumbled as he slurped.

Eric told me he was changing his name. "Amaranth!" he announced. He said it with passion. He said it with flair. He told me that it wasn't only a beautiful flower, but it also meant "everlasting." A symbolic name to match his desires: Eric Amaranth wanted to have good, healthy orgasms forevermore. We finally had something in common. We both wanted to extend our not-yet-dead time, only I preferred to preserve myself with bottles of wine rather than turn into a living compost with his diet of vegetables and protein shakes.

Naked. He had me on my back. He went under the hood, checking up on my orgasm gear. We worked the Saber and dildo in tandem again. "Get it right on the clit there," he said of my

Saber placement, as he bobbed the pink dildo in and out. "Good."

Then he asked if I'd allow him to taste the twinkle.

I thought for a while. "No," I said.

"Pleasure reluctance?" he inquired. And then he asked me how I had come to my negative conclusion.

He had stumped me; I realized that I'd answered no simply out of habit.

"Yes," I said, amending my previous response. "Try her out."

He explained, as a good teacher would, that if we adhered to the strictest and safest sex regulations, he *should* be using a dental dam. Lesson learned for next time. He went down past my bellybutton and stopped at the crook where my legs met. He didn't quite fit, so his excess self ended up cramped up against my dresser. Every once in a while, I heard tchotchkes knock over. It didn't matter. This was my first real oral examination, experimentation, exploration, with possible side effects of extreme excitation. My legs quivered. But then I looked down and lost my concentration. I saw only Eric's eyes, the rest of his face disappearing below my pubic hair. From my vantage point, the unwieldy black, wiry mess hovering below Eric's nose reminded me of my romantic interest—Hank's beard.

I was feeling bad about Hank; he was probably hard at work, recording something in his studio, while I was with a sacred whore. Then I began feeling bad that I wasn't having a good old-fashioned M & J orgasm. Everyone always told me that this—going down on Clitty—would be the no-questions-asked path to coming, but Clitty Rose wasn't having any of it. Orgasm continued to mystify her while in anyone else's company but mine.

"No orgasm," I reported.

"But does it feel good?" Eric said, lifting his head for a second.

And it did. Come to think of it—sensationally—it felt awesome.

THE PUSSY WHISPERER WOULD LIKE ALL WOMEN

"Yeah," I said. "Amazing."

Amaranth dove back in. He was like David Blaine, he was down there so long. About a half hour later, he came up for a breather. He looked at me, with hungry wide eyes. Pussy was obviously the fuel he ran on. It was his Red Bull. He lingered between my legs a little longer. He was thinking something. His eyes were rotating somewhere in the nether regions of my ceiling.

"I probably shouldn't even ask this," he said.

Is he going to hang me from the ceiling?

"I can probably guess," he continued, "but have you ever had anyone go down on your ass?"

I clamped my legs together. I got up on my elbows. I looked at him like he was an alien. "No," I said. "Really, my ass? You want to go down on my *ass*?"

I'd totally missed the ass-eating memo.

"Yeah," he said, leaning on his forearms at the foot of the bed. "Wash up, soap and water."

I thought about Q-tips and my orgasmic ears, and figured there could be a million other untapped spots on my body that could turn me inside out with pleasure. The cooter is great, but I suppose it's not *all* about her. I breathed. The butt. The butt, it's the responsible thing to do.

I washed up quickly, thankfully not running into Leigh or Ursula in the hallway. Amaranth rolled me onto my stomach. He told me the butt was highly underrated. He wished men weren't so afraid of the ass, like it somehow always had to be homoerotic. "There's nothing much hotter than a masculine man getting strap-on butt-fucked," he said, trying to set the record straight.

I breathed and breathed again. I stuffed my face into a pillow. My eyes wanted to roll back, but I took them around with me as I twisted my body to see what was happening back there, what was creating this sensation like none I'd ever had before. Flickers of feeling wound around my torso. It tickled, it hurt, it scratched, it made me want to undulate, then collapse.

My butt was being enlightened. My butt was happy. My butt was in nirvana. My butt was angry I'd gone twenty-six years without doing this before. I wanted to send this memo out. I wanted to spam everyone's in-boxes with it. I wanted everyone to get their asses gnawed on at some point. The world would be better for it.

Then my phone rang. While Eric was in mid-lick, I looked at the screen. It said Hank. Hank. I hung up. I hung up on Hank while I was getting my ass eaten out by a sacred whore.

I felt kind of weird about that.

Eric was at my side now. I helped him come. He even complimented me while I was pleasuring him. "Your hand looks cute," he said, "the way it's wrapped around."

And he must be pretty damn healthy because his orgasm, I was pretty sure, reverberated all the way to Manhattan. On that day, it wasn't the subway rumbling underground, it was the bass of his roaring. I didn't know whether to throw a pillow over his mouth or record the sound and play it over and over again. The next morning, Leigh asked me with a panicked look if everything was okay.

"What do you mean?" I asked.

"It sounded like a cow was slaughtered in your room last night," she said.

"No," I said, laughing, "that was just Amaranth getting off."

Eric gave me a peck. If we frenched, I'd be worried that if he opened his mouth all the way, his lips would encompass my entire head. He'd swallow me. He ran his fingers through my hair.

I asked him if he would ever go monogamous. He said it wouldn't be fair to all the ladies. He said he was like a chocolate cake; most men were perfunctory-type desserts like Oreos. It took effort to be decadent. "Every straight girl should have one of me," he said. "The only problem is, there is only one of me."

I was thinking, Wow, he thinks he's God's gift to women. But you know what? He's probably right. He believed that women deserved every single ounce of respect and care he gave them.

He told me that he wanted me to find a man with his spirit. "Someone who's slow," he said. "Every woman deserves time and patience. Strokes can be infinite."

Maybe I'd found that, I thought.

You can't move much more slowly than Hank and me.

I felt like I had to tell Hank about everything I was doing with Eric. I guess I did feel a bit guilty. I wish I was better at lying, but I kept being reminded of what I'd done. There was even a report card—Eric's critique on my masturbatory performance—in my inbox the following morning.

Eric "Amaranth" Wilkinson to me:

i think if you try stroking the vibe over your clitoris, like a finger sort of, that combined with the vibe will do better for you and creates variation in the sensation so you may not have to stop and rest her. You could also try a higher speed and lightly touch the vibe tip to your clit and then move it around the glans like a fingertip. But i think, from what i saw last night, you may be leaving it in one spot with not enough vibe power and it's not the right stimulation for her.

kiss! —*Eric*

I wanted Hank to understand the educational value, so I took him out for a glass of wine to talk about—while also hopefully taking the edge off—the issue.

"I have to tell you the truth," I said. "I was with a sacred whore last Tuesday."

His brows folded forward so far they were acting like secondary eyelids. His eyes were slits.

"But it wasn't romantic," I said. "It's educational. My sacred whore is actually the boyfriend of the Mother of Masturbation. So, you see, it doesn't mean anything. Really."

"What does sacred whore mean exactly?" he asked.

"Well," I said, "he gives me options and I choose what I want." He didn't look pleased, but on some level he was accepting.

"What if I call him a sex surrogate," I said. "Is that better?"

"That just means whore with different words," he said. "Doesn't it?"

"Kind of," I said.

He said he'd be okay with it until we were monogamous. (At that point, he didn't want me needing a merkin to hide uninvited bacteria, from my meandering, into the bedroom.)

But monogamy scared me. It did. It was like the M-word made people go out and do ludicrous things. Look at Eliot Spitzer—he was monogamous and wound up as Client 9.

Sometimes it seemed that monogamy was invented just to corner people into cheating. If there was no monogamy, there could be no cheating. It's a construct that seems to punish one half when the other half gets the urge, which many biologists say is inevitable; it's in our blood to pilfer outside crotches. People smoked cigarettes, thinking they looked cool, for a long time before doctors discovered they caused cancer. Monogamy, too, has been practiced for quite a while. I'm just saying.

Hank quickly became more concerned about other things.

"This is so weird," he said. "You're probably going to write this conversation in the book. Aren't you? Right now, this. People will

THE PUSSY WHISPERER WOULD LIKE ALL WOMEN

read this. They'll know that you saw a sacred whore while I was with you and I stayed with you. My friends will think I'm an idiot. I'm continuing to see a girl who has a sacred whore. You see? It's weird."

"Yeah," I said, "it's a little different, but tell me this: Have you ever gotten your ass eaten out before?"

ANGINA GOFER MOMS

It was around this time that I got a call from OneTaste about a possible interview with Nicole Daedone. Yes, The Gasm was finally ready for me. I'd been asking, and had been denied, for the past six months now. I hadn't been back to their center for months, but I'd received calls asking me to go to events. They'd rattle off long pitches, weaving in and out of sex-speak, as if it were all typed up in a manual, like the lines call-center operators regurgitate while working a fundraiser. And like telemarketers, no matter what time of day they called, they always seemed to catch me during dinner.

I wasn't sure about it. I appreciated what OneTaste was about—their ideas, their openness, the way they were truly helping people with sex and life—so it was hard to understand why they turned me off. Maybe it was the push-pull thing; they seemed to want me to join so bad that I had a Groucho Marx–like reaction: "I would not join any club that would have someone like me as a member." (That is, of course, unless it offered subsidized health coverage.)

Maybe I saw them as a capitalist encroachment on the crotch—
orgasm gone franchise. They have two centers now and hope to
open more. What if they patented the orgasm and women of the
world would have to pay royalties each time our uteruses contracted? When I talked to a high-ranking member in San Francisco, he said his desire for the future was that every Starbucks
would offer a fifteen-minute twat tickle while you waited for your
latte. He also said there was a prevailing feeling in the world: Kill
what you can't fuck. Hence, less killing if you had more fucking.
"There'd be less war," he said.

I had to admit, I liked the sound of that. Maybe I was just jealous I wasn't capitalizing on orgasm myself. Oops, wait, maybe I
was. Never mind.

I'd brought up my ambivalence with OneTaste to Rori. She said
I should probably just listen to myself. She said sex is listening to
your desire. "It's what works for you," she'd said. "Don't let everyone dump what they think sex is into you."

But despite my feelings—whatever they were—I still maintained
this nebulous fascination with OneTaste's founder. I'd heard even
more stories since San Francisco. The Gasm had been mute for a
year straight two separate times. That's a cumulative two years of
saying nothing. Silence always made people seem wiser (I should
take note of that). She'd also written two full books in less than two
months—just channeling words through her fingertips. Even Zola,
who was impervious to most encounters, got fazed after talking to
The Gasm.

From the beginning of my journey, I got stuck with this idea
that Ms. Daedone was the one to tell me the MEANING OF OR-
GASM. So after the call notifying me that she might be available,
I frantically exchanged e-mails with her assistant—not giving them

an extra second to renege on my opportunity. We worked out logistics.

I told myself I wasn't going to be anxious. So what if she could read minds? So what if she'd managed to lecture me in my unconscious? So what if tear ducts became open spigots in her presence? So what if people stopped in their tracks the moment they spotted a lone Perrier bottle, a signal of her impending arrival? I was going to remain relaxed.

The day I was supposed to meet her, I got three text messages, each telling me to meet in a different location. When I finally reached the destination, I got another text that said she'd just left and would meet me back at OneTaste headquarters. How rude, I thought. But when I arrived, I acted graciously to her assistant. I quickly scanned my notebook, where I'd jotted down questions, as she led me up a flight of stairs to another sparsely decorated room—wood floors, white walls, and a blue sofa with The Gasm sitting languidly on it.

The assistant shut the door. The Gasm and I were finally alone. I lowered my ass into an adjacent chair as she assessed me. My heart thumped in my gut.

I thought I'd hit her with a shocker. I figured she'd respect someone who was a truth-teller. I told her that I didn't know why, but I felt repelled by OneTaste even though I admired all their teachings.

She shifted, put one foot under her tush. Her arms were spread across the back of the couch. She knocked her ponytail back and forth like a horse swatting a fly from its back and set her chin up, before releasing a statement.

"If you can go away," she said, "then go away. If someone can't enter, then that's good, I trust."

So much for starting with a shocker. Her response knocked me off what little game I'd brought with me. A good cult wouldn't acquiesce so easily to defectors. Shouldn't it fight to get as many members as it could?

Then I blanked.

"Nice pomegranates," I said, pointing to the bowl on the coffee table.

"Yeah," she said. "I was just admiring the arrangement; it's beautiful."

For the next thirty-seven minutes, I somehow managed to stay mostly conscious while she kept the conversation going. Her hand movements hypnotized me; they were like a hula dance on an acid trip.

I said bye as soon as it seemed like an appropriate-length interview to warrant six months of waiting.

"There's no rush," she said.

She was nice. She was smart. She believed in orgasm.

"I know you're busy," I said and rushed the door, clomped down the stairs until I reached the fresh air. When I came bumbling onto the street with a vertigo-enhanced scowl, frustrated that I'd let her reputation fluster me, the only thing that stayed with me was that she said orgasm gave people direct access to the way things were.

If so, orgasm was telling me the interview was a disaster.

As I walked, I called Zola. I asked if she could meet me for a coffee. I was feeling vexed from my counter-serendipitous momentary loss of volition. I hadn't asked The Gasm the looming question. I hadn't asked her about the MEANING OF ORGASM. Zola said she'd be a little while. "Girl! I'm doing my taxes," she said. "I'm the only sex worker I know who files."

I meandered toward the Greenmarket to visit with Atman. He could give me solace, even if it was ephemeral. But then Fiona came to mind. She thought she'd find answers by going to India, that mystical place. Gurus grew like weeds out there. Yoga was born there. Siddhartha sat under a banyan tree there and, bam, he turned into Buddha. Enlightenment. Nirvana. Something more. (And hopefully a lot of good souvenir shopping.)

But she'd sent me a few e-mail missives in the past two weeks. India wasn't meeting her expectations. She hated it there. She wanted to leave early. India was dirty, she said, litter was everywhere. She said there was no organization; it was chaos. She was disillusioned. There were more white people in her yoga classes there than in the ones she attended in New York. (She seemed to think brown people made experiences authentic—but was that why I kept seeking out my guru of crotch?) She'd spent more than a grand on an airline ticket to find answers, and there were only more questions.

Even though I wanted a scone, I didn't stop by Atman's stall. I didn't want to be tempted to lay my dilemma into someone else's hands like I always seemed to do.

Then again, there I was with Zola. She licked latte foam from her finger. "Yuuummm," she groaned. She wasn't in her usual attire; she'd selected a red hoodie, which matched her crimson lipstick. She looked like a Geisha meets Compton style. I told her The Gasm's mythology had bungled my cool during the interview. Zola told me to look on the bright side. She reminded me that I could deduct all my vibrators as work-related expenses. Then she told me to buy a butt plug, a little one, and remember to keep the receipt for next year's write-offs. "It opens up the first chakra," she said of the butt plug, "and releases tension."

When I got home, I was pulsating with caffeine. I sat down with THE MEANING OF ORGASM typed on a blank screen. What *did* it mean? I'd been thinking of it all wrong. I realized it didn't have to be in capitals. So I took it out of caps lock—meaning of orgasm—and then scrambled it around. I made anagrams.

> meaning of orgasm
> enraging oaf moms
> mafia monger song
> managing some fro
> angina gofer moms
> mania gnome frogs
> anemia from gongs
> mama fingers goon
> fireman gags moon
> fame aging morons
> safe man grooming
> enigma farms goon
> mega morning sofa

Depending on how you looked at it, the meaning of orgasm could be many different things.

GOOD

Hank and I went out to dinner. I think I knew unconsciously, maybe even a tad bit consciously, that it was going to happen. I showered, I shaved, and even put effort toward smelling good. I also dropped an extra pair of contact lenses into my purse—one-day disposables—just in case.

I was looking at him across the table. I got a glimpse of that corneal acceptance he'd offered me before, while we were in the horizontal. I kept thinking I liked him, but why did I like him? Why him? But it was *him*.

"Do you have commitment issues?" I asked him.

We were doing Hand Kama Sutra over the table—holding, grabbing, intertwining, tickling, caressing each other's palms.

"I might have some," he said. "Do you?"

"I think I do," I said.

"Everyone has some commitment issues."

"Maybe we should get rid of commitment so people could have less issues," I said.

I had visited with Rori earlier in the week. She wasn't wearing her usual knee-high boots, just strappy heels, her ankles showing. Must have been spring in the air. We were all steadily getting a little more naked as the Earth warmed.

I told her I was having problems getting close to Hank.

"Hank's kind," I said. "He's great. But he has a gut. A belly."

She propped her elbows on the armrests and clasped her fingers together. Nodded for me to elaborate.

"It's not about looks," I said. "It's about longevity. He can't go running with me."

She continued nodding.

"We could never last together," I said. "His house is too messy."

I stared out the window. I was really on a roll.

"He's ticklish," I said. "I can't even touch him."

I cocked my head to the side.

"Have you heard of beard dandruff?"

She had a smirk as she ran a hand through her hair. She never wore it up. Even psychologists needed something to fidget with.

She told me that concentrating on those characteristics was just a method of distancing myself, making myself feel safe, convincing myself it would never work out as I'd done by choosing emotionally unavailable men or ones on different continents in the past.

"It's great," she said.

"What do you mean?" I said. "There are problems; it's not working out."

"You're still with him," she said. "Focusing on those things is allowing you to stay, to make it seem impermanent."

"So what does that mean?" I said. "If I stay with him, I'm always going to be tearing him apart."

"We'll work on that later," she said. "I'm just happy you're enjoying someone, that you're getting intimate."

I'm despicable. I appreciated someone only through some sort of emotional sadism. It was true that I'd been focusing on the negatives, but maybe Rori was right because meanwhile I didn't want to go to sleep without giving him a call first to say good night. I saw things in stores and made mental notes of what he might want. I even baked him a banana cake with the density he liked: the thickness of my quadriceps. He'd seeped into me despite my self-preservational compulsion to discount him.

And here he was now, in front of me, trying to determine the sexual orientation of our tableside neighbors.

"Bi," he said.

"Definitely gay," I countered.

We went to his apartment and watched *Michael Clayton*. And every once in a while we would kiss. And then watch and then kiss again. And I was thinking George Clooney is hot. Hank is not George Clooney, I thought. But that didn't matter because I liked Hank.

It was too much for us when George caught Tilda Swinton red-handed. It was so cathartic we ripped our clothes off—well, as soon as Hank complied and turned off the light switch. He seized my shirt. My bra, I unhooked. His shirt, I don't know where it went. We kissed. I kept getting beard hairs in my mouth. And I'd pinch around on my tongue, trying to fish them out.

"There's a lot more where that came from," he said, as I flicked it.

We went to his bedroom. I used his laundry pile as a ladder to climb up to his mattress. We rolled around. I steamrolled him, going up one side of his belly and over the edge of the other. Zola had recently begun dating a guy with a protruding belly, too. She told me the belly was actually a blessing as it served much better than flat stomachs to grind on—it wasn't a stomach, it was a clit-grinding mound—which made orgasms all the more likely during sex.

Hank's warmth felt good. He was so close to me. There was a vacuum between my legs. I wanted to suck him up it.

I stopped moving, pushed his shoulder up a little. I looked into his eyes. He took off his glasses. I didn't want to be inappropriate. I didn't want to assume things. I cleared my throat.

"If we were to desire to have sex," I said, "would you happen to have a condom?"

"If we did choose to have sex," he said, "yes, I would happen to have a condom."

He didn't move. He still wasn't moving. Why wasn't he moving?

"Okay, get one!"

He put it over the tip; I helped him roll it down. I told him we had to start with missionary; I wasn't ready to be the rhythmically responsible one. He hovered above me in push-up position—I saw how he worked now; his idea of exercise occurred only in the bedroom. This was the type of guy who had to be sexercised regularly. I held his potbelly, like a globe, in my hands.

"I'm Atlas," I said, smiling.

Then he lowered down.

"I'm inside you," he said.

"No, I'm enveloping you," I said.

And then came the noises of sex. The heavy breathing, the crumpling of a condom, the suction of fluids, and I thought this should be a fucking CD—a fucking CD of fucking—this should be a soundtrack to something, and it was: to our evening.

And he had rhythm. He'd done this before. Hank was my number six and a half. Oh fuck it, who am I kidding: I'm fine with seven now.

I was finally part of the conversation downstairs. I wasn't listening to the droning of my brain's mundane monologue. I pictured my clit swimming up and lodging itself into the middle of my forehead, an illustration of symbiosis—the crotch-brain connection at its finest. I wasn't sidetracked, worrying about Hank getting me somewhere, because I already knew how to do it on my own. I think Betty would call this having found my foundation. Self-sufficient with my sensations. By not depending on Hank and freeing him from my expectations, I could actually be even closer to him. I was completely there. Moment to moment. Taking it in like I never had before.

And I laughed. I laughed harder. I felt good about laughing. We looked at each other. He asked why I was laughing.

I said, "Hey, just let me laugh."

And then he came. These grunts expelling into my ear canal, coming into two canals at once. It was like the biggest fattest hottest Q-tip was up in there, dangerously digging toward my brain. Shivers rocketed from my lobe to my nether regions and back up again. I'm still eargasmic! There is a sensation hierarchy and ears do not hold the crown—they're no traditional orgasm for sure—but if you ask me, that's pleasure. My shoulders jutted upward from sparking nerves and my eyes closed as Hank rolled off. I got my pleasure; pleasure comes in myriad forms.

He lay beside me and I felt wetness on my body. I was lying in a puddle. I blamed it on him. "Did you pee?" I said, joking.

He said it was me.

"*Me?*" I said.

Then I remembered that horrifically vivid video about female ejaculation. Could I have . . . no. Had I?

Maybe I had.

And I smiled to myself.

GOOD

Well, whatever the lagoon's origins, I tried to avoid its shore as we cuddled. The wind whipped; I could hear it against the window. Cars were honking down below. And even though we were intertwined, looking like one globular form, I didn't feel diminished. I wasn't suddenly Mar or Ra—I still felt whole, Mara. He'd managed to snuggle my entirety. Only add to me. Meanwhile the people outside were yelping to express their surplus of partying. It was a Thursday night before Good Friday. And I thought, How is it that "Good" is used as an adjective to commemorate the day someone was crucified? Then Hank fell asleep. Snores started up. I kicked him. The snores stopped. And I thought this, this I could call Good.

UNVEILING

Two months later, I found myself wearing a cotton gown that went down to my knees and tied loosely in the back, with nothing underneath. My clammy feet stuck slightly to the linoleum as I teetered back and forth. The woman in front of me, clad in a lab coat, had a bright orange magnet the size of a small anvil in one hand and my hot-pink veiny dildo in the other. She was checking it for metal. She told me no metal was allowed inside the fMRI. I'd once read an article that described how someone accidentally brought an oxygen tank into an fMRI room and it flew so fast toward the machine that it killed someone in the midst of its trajectory. I instantly concocted horrific visuals of deadly flying dildos.

I had nerves. My nerves were in full force. I shouldn't be nervous though. Just a month ago I had Clitty Rose photographed. I got my own private pornography done, like Fiona was always telling me to do. She'd said I'd love my body if I saw it through an artist's eyes. I wanted to challenge myself and got all worked up about the shoot the week before, but when the photographer, Andrew Brucker, came over for our session, I easily whipped off my clothes and deemed it more of a celebration. No nerves there. My rib cage was jutting out due to an extreme arc and twist of the back that Brucker was trying to capture. It was uncomfortable, not because of my nudity but because I was developing a cramp. I even held still while he covered my little butt boil with makeup. Ursula told me lots of exfoliation would get rid of that, but exfoliation was painful. "We can't have that," he'd said.

Blemishes don't exist on film. They don't; I won't ever expect them to.

When Fiona returned from India, I showed her the photos. She pointed at the screen and covered her mouth with her other hand. "Mar!" she said. "I didn't even let him shoot me at that angle!"

"I went more nudie than *you*?" I said, flabbergasted. We had broken our roles. I kind of wished she had told me that she hadn't gone open-beaver for the photographer before I'd done the shoot, but you know what? Fuck it. Clitty Rose deserved her close-up after all she'd been through. I wasn't even too embarrassed (okay, I was kind of) when Brucker said he hadn't seen one as bushy as mine in more than a decade. "The girls take it all off these days," he'd said, noting how popular it is for girls to try to pretend like they're not mammals. "That's the style." I guess I'm a late bloomer, still. I don't keep up with the latest crotch fashion.

But this situation was different. My jitters, I determined, were appropriate. Four researchers, including Dr. Komisaruk, watched as this lab-coat-clad woman manhandled my phallus. My appliances were out for everyone to see. I never thought I'd be showing them off in public like that. All I'd have to do is tell them all to sniff it, and I'd practically be Betty.

The woman led me into the fMRI room. She laid me flat on the gurney and pulled a thin sheet over my body. She locked my head into place with a cage-looking device. I was restrained. My feet were facing the glass window, which separated me from Dr.

Komisaruk and his three assistants. They could see me clearly from the control room. They could see everything I was about to do.

She tucked my gadgets—my lube and dildo—near my hands. I wondered if Dr. Komisaruk would find the "I" that made "me" today. I'd asked him earlier, "Did you find out where is I?"

"We're still looking," he replied.

I wasn't surprised. That "I" is a sneaky little bugger, more elusive than any orgasm ever was.

My coping mechanisms were getting a big workout. They were in fifth gear now. I smiled the kind of smile only clowns seem to achieve when using paint to go outside normal lip bounds. I was about to masturbate in front of scientists while being restrained—exhibitionism at its most sterile, with a tinge of BDSM.

Over dinner a week before, Dr. Komisaruk had told me that the primary importance of the fMRI would be to map the vulva structure in my brain. It hasn't been done yet. There are maps for the hand, the leg, the face, and even the penis, which is all laid out in a diagram by Dr. Wilder Penfield. Unsurprisingly, the medical establishment has ignored our pussies. Dr. Komisaruk said I'd be asked to stimulate my clit, vaginal canal, and then cervix to see which areas respectively sparked in my brain. Then I'd have ten minutes to try to work myself up to a climax. I'd have to raise my hand as a signal when I finally made it to orgasm—*if* I made it to orgasm, that is.

As the fMRI appointment approached, I'd had a session with Rori.

"Don't worry so much about the orgasm," she said. "It's not about the goal, it's about the journey."

"I know," I said. "I get it, but that's just such a cliché."

"Clichés are clichés for a reason," she said.

"But it's for science," I said. "I have to orgasm for science!"

UNVEILING

The assistant pressed some sort of button on the side of the fMRI and I started sliding inside. They told me it would be claustrophobic. I had said I wasn't claustrophobic, but then I *was*: It was like someone had lodged my head into a toilet paper roll. It felt lonely in there. But then Dr. Komisaruk spoke up: I could hear his voice through my headphones. It was nice to have company. He was the master of ceremonies. He told me to prepare for mapping. I had an hour and a half of mapping in front of me before I could go free-style.

The machine started. It sounded like a digitalized version of a jackhammer. For some reason, while in that toilet paper roll, I thought of The Collector's hoard. The pile hasn't changed since he started with his pills, but through its stagnation, his pile of junk has fermented into something more. It's produced seedlings—we have plants blossoming out of the backyard garbage dump. And I think that's pretty special, even if they are just messy weeds working their way up, ineptly and haphazardly through a sea of black plastic. Because I can relate: I feel like I'm growing, but in a messy, haphazard, somewhat inept way too.

It's not necessarily something that can be helped, this ineptitude. I get it now; humans have just been dealt an immense number of annoying and inefficient emotions to deal with life.

That knowledge takes adjusting to.

I'm still unsure about a lot of things, including the role that Hank plays in my life. When I told my mom that I still wasn't sure about him, she had one quick retort.

"Mara," she said, "he's the only one who's managed to fuck you in a year. That means something."

That shut me up for a bit.

I think I was half sleeping because when Dr. Komisaruk's voice came through and said it was time for free-style, my hand charged into my vulva without me allowing it to.

I feared my sheet would fall off, but then I realized I was way more naked than nudity: these scientists were seeing what was inside me. This was as intimate as it got. They were seeing my mortality, my carnality, my sexuality, my humanity—my lumpy, bulbous brain. My crotch would be sparking in my cortex on a big screen. Dr. Komisaruk and his assistants, if all went well, would be watching me make live-action brain pornography.

One of Dr. Komisaruk's research partners, Nan Wise, came in and lubed up my dildo because being inside this toilet paper roll, I couldn't see anything. I was dependent on them for everything. Now I had the slippery rod in my hand. My ten minutes were already counting down. I gave the dildo no other options but to be shoved up my insides. The jackhammering gave me a rhythm. The sheet was getting caught; it was distracting. *I'm not going to come*, I thought, and I thought I'd refund them the one hundred dollars they had paid me to be a research subject. Zola had been so excited about the cash, too. "You're a sex worker!" she'd shouted. All the scientists were watching me. I could envision them at the window. I started thinking I had to get out of there and go somewhere. We'd discussed this compulsion before, Rori and me.

"Where do you have to go?" she'd asked.

I don't know.

"What would it be like to stay?"

Is there any such thing as staying? I ask.

I feel myself tightening up. I'm flexing all my muscles. Dr. Komisaruk had told me that, counter to what some other researchers have found, during orgasm, the brain is lit up like few other activities—it's more alive than ever. No *le petit mort*. I'm in darkness, but my brain must be a light show because I'm starting to feel the buildup. I'm stirring, and pinching, and stroking the strokes the Orgasm People taught me, but I'm also preparing for a crotch sneeze. I don't want to ask for too much. And my hand starts to tentatively rise. My hand is now stretched all the way into the air to signal the oncoming of my come. My faculties must be magnetic, because the machine is unhinging them. They've never sprung apart like this before. My vagina is high-fiving the dildo over and over again. These contractions are much more than a handshake— it keeps clamping down. My uterine contractions aren't embarrassed about my dildo's hot-pink gaudiness. She's not as superficial as I am—she seems to like it just fine. All the while, I don't make a sound. My hand in the air says all there is to say. Maybe I'm just a sexual mute. That's liberation, too. And then my hand surrenders, lowering down as my body relaxes. I feel in love with this machine. What a great piece of metal.

The jackhammering of the machine stops. The assistant presses a button, which slides me out. My hair is shooting out in all directions like something feral and unkempt. The sheets are twisted around my legs. My eyes are groggy; I rub them like I've woken up from hibernation. I'd like to be humping Hank's legs right now, and clawing at his back, like the cats at home do my periwinkle sofa. Then I sit up, a bit woozy. In the window facing me, the four researchers stand side by side—Dr. Komisaruk in the middle— applauding.

I swing my feet to the ground and pad, dildo in hand, around the corner to central command. I spot my bulbous brain, the membrane that makes me me, on the screen in 3-D. I'm a brain porn star. Barry sidles up to me—not at all put off by the gooey oblong object that keeps threatening to slip out of my grasp—and pats me on the back. "Way to go, kiddo," he says, smiling.

I smile back. I love a happy ending.

ACKNOWLEDGMENTS

A big fat thank you goes out to all the sex educators and academics who agreed so enthusiastically to help me in my orgasmic mission— Eric Amaranth, Barry Komisaruk, Nan Wise, Eleni Frangos, Betty Dodson, Tallulah Sulis, Dorrie Lane, Barbara Carrellas, Satya, Annie Sprinkle, Carol Queen, R.J. Noonan, Barry Goldman, and OneTaste. Their insights and counsel changed my life (and those of everyone else they touch) for the more pleasurable. Special thanks to the Orgasm People for their generous scholarship and for teaching me concepts that will echo in my brain, at the most intimate of moments, for the remainder of my days. Thanks to Jim Abraham, Andrew Brucker, Will Baxter, and Brian McDermott for their generosity. Larry Seiler showed me how to be brave. Thanks to the Brooklyn Library for books (I swear I'll return them soon). Zola is the Mother Theresa of sex workers. Her charity and perspective inspired me (and thanks for the Chakra tonings). Thank you to Vanessa Gould, Emma Span, Nora Weinberg, Denise Carson, Rori, Leigh, Judy Altman, Louise Rothman, Karen Kashkin, Atman, Haresh Bhojwani, and Rafiq for their encouragement and input. Thanks to my editor, Rakesh Satyal, at HarperCollins for taking a risk on me, trusting me, letting me go nuts . . . and then editing me. Rob Crawford over there too! I'm grateful to my agent, Chris Parris-Lamb, for his edits, ideas, support, and belief, and for returning my I'm-freaking-out phone calls (though I'm still wondering when he's going to deliver those chill pills he told me to take). Thanks to Prospect Park, the Brooklyn Bridge, India, Cusco, Bangkok, my windowsill, the periwinkle sofa, and perfectly twisted dollops of nondairy soft-serve for provoking endless thought. Thanks to Hank for telling me not to negotiate with book terrorists, even though he was one of them. And more importantly, I thank him for continuing to talk to me even after he read the book. I'm grateful for twenty years and counting of Fiona. I couldn't have done this without her 24-hour help line. Thanking David Blum times infinity doesn't even seem like enough. He was the first person to take me seriously as a writer among a trillion other things. So, thank you times infinity squared (cubed?). And then there's my family who I'd like to thank profusely for not disowning me. I have much gratitude for my grandparents, who not only embraced the writing of this book but also agreed to share their own story. Thanks to my brothers, Matt and Logan, for making fun of me only half the time (I know it tool a lot of restraint). And lastly, thanks to my parents. Without their love, support, and acceptance (not to mention their gametes), this book would not even have been attemptable.

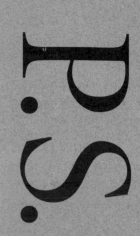

About the author

About the book

Read on

Insights,
Interviews
& More . . .

An Interview with My Flour Baby Daddy (FBD)

In my junior high school sex education course, my classmates and I had to form pairs and switch off carrying around five-pound sacks of flour. Caring for the flour sacks was supposed to simulate the trials and tribulations of caring for human babies, thereby discouraging us from engaging in any baby-making activities. Twelve years after that project, I reunited with my former partner—who I refer to here as my Flour Baby Daddy—over the Internet. To examine the long-term impact of our sex education, I chose to conduct an interview with him over ichat. The following interview is a condensed, edited, and slightly altered version of that interview.

  me: hey!
 FBD: hey you!
  me: Now good for the interview?
 FBD: yeah, sounds good.
  me: so i'm going to interview you about being my flour baby daddy and how our junior high abstinence-based sex education program affected you. so do you remember doing flour babies?
 FBD: only since you reminded me of it. Hehehe.
        "come on baby, knead that dough!"
  me: when you are reminded of flour babies, what do you remember?
 FBD: I remember that the one thing about them was how awkward it was to be carrying around a thing of flour. it really didn't help shape my thoughts towards anything at all.
  me: so even though they were called flour babies, you didn't think of them as babies?

FBD: it may have just been how i was
brought up (catholic family that
believes in birth control), but i never
had any need to care for a "baby."

me: like you weren't worried that if you had
sex, you might have to end up carrying
around a five-pound sack of milled
grain?

FBD: no, i didn't.

me: how would you describe who you were
in high school?

FBD: heh, i was an uptight arrogant band
nerd who didn't get along with many
people . . . but tried to do so anyways

me: :)
that's why I didn't want to be your
flour baby mommy. Did you know
I didn't want to be your flour baby
mommy? It wasn't the band nerd
part, but the anger mean part.

FBD: :: nods
i've grown past that. i chalk it up to
teenage angst

me: i think you threatened me with a
ruptured flour baby, powdered innards
everywhere.

FBD: what!? what is this slander you sling
about ;0
K, i may have, unfortunately :(
honestly, i dont remember the details
of your/our interaction with the flour
baby

me: :(
Then do you remember egg
babies?

FBD: yup, we did those in "decision making"
our freshman year.

me: so what do you think is better, egg
babies or flour babies?

FBD: they are both yet another waste of class
time.

me: FBD, please answer the question.
Which one? ▶

An Interview with My Flour Baby Daddy (FBD) *(continued)*

FBD: hmm. flour babies do a great job of showing how awkward it is to carry around a 5 lb sack of whatever, but the egg babies are def more fragile. though, you can easily stick the flour in a backpack/locker and let it suffocate through the day.

me: true.

FBD: hard to do that with an egg . . . hmm . . . did you know anyone that hardboiled their eggs? I guess I'm still undecided between eggs and flour.

me: okay, instead of carrying around baked goods, what would you have liked to learn in sex ed?
(my armpits reek right now)

FBD: myself, I would have rather learned more about sex. what women like, what pleases them, how to be gentle :P
(that's why they have this thing called deodorant)

me: how did you figure it all out then—you know, assuming you figured it out—if our teachers only gave us products for pastries?
(I don't like to use it)

FBD: if anything, it helped me be more curious about things.
the lack of information made me want to know what i was missing.
(then don't complain)

me: okay, say carrying around groceries and pretending they were babies actually did manage to deter adolescents from sex, which grocery item would have stopped you?
(asshole)

FBD is offline. ∾

Reading Comprehension and More

1. What did I often purchase from Atman?
   A. French maid uniforms
   B. Spanish and Swahili translations of the Kama Sutra
   C. Carrot-raisin scones
   D. Double-headed dildos

2. Hank had . . .
   A. A perpetual piece of parsley stuck between his front teeth
   B. Beard dandruff
   C. A voice that sounded like an ice machine
   D. A phobia of Wondrous Vulva Puppets with Peruvian tapestry-covered labias

3. Fiona has . . .
   A. Always felt this way before
   B. Would like to feel this way again
   C. Has never felt this way before
   D. Likes the way that this way feels

4. My grandpa . . .
   A. Collects different editions of *Gone With the Wind*
   B. Sculpts nudes
   C. Has been known to go for golf cart joy rides
   D. Went to Israel and became enamored with his tour guide, Omer

5. After Hank read the book, he . . .
   A. Began using Head and Shoulders on his beard
   B. Still insisted he had a third testicle
   C. Told me I had a girl-stache
   D. Wouldn't friend me on Facebook ▶

Reading Comprehension and More
(continued)

6. After reading the book, Rori, my therapist . . .
   A. Took off one of her high heels and lobbed it at my head
   B. Asked if I was sure I didn't want to take her up on the twice-a-week sessions
   C. Asked what I thought she'd thought about when she read the book
   D. Admitted that she should see a therapist about her Diet Peach Snapple problem

7. Carl collects . . .
   A. Oyster shells
   B. Heaps of trash
   C. Socks that have strayed from their pairs
   D. Pictures of women's armpits

8. When I asked Atman if he was okay with using his real name in the book, he said . . .
   A. You want to know more about your flower?
   B. Nice day, isn't it?
   C. The book is neurological with your psychology
   D. Atman is Atman

9. Buddy, Sika, and Lucy . . .
   A. Are what I named Hank's three testicles
   B. Are my roommate's three cats
   C. Are what Atman calls his disciples
   D. All of the above

10. Eric, my sacred whore, changed his last name from Wilkinson to . . .
    A. Sacred Whore
    B. Artichoke
    C. Amaranth
    D. Saffron

11. What does Zola often do when she eats?
    A. Pukes in order to maintain her figure
    B. Stops, drops, and rolls
    C. Just says "No"
    D. Shudders and moans

12. What did women at some of the go-go bars in Bangkok shoot out of their vulvas?
    A. Stuffed elephants named Earl
    B. Ping-Pong balls
    C. Beard dandruff
    D. Ant tattoos

13. My sacred whore gave me a vibrator called . . .
    A. Curious George
    B. The Darth Invader
    C. The Saber
    D. The Little Engine That Could

14. Tallulah, in the Native American Choctaw language, means . . .
    A. Crouching tiger
    B. Hidden dragon
    C. Leaping water
    D. Spanakopita

15. Barry Komisaruk makes D.I.Y. dildos out of . . .
    A. Plexiglas rods
    B. Twenty-five-inch walrus baculums
    C. Bicycle seats
    D. Diet Peach Snapple bottles

Answers: 1: C. 2: B. 3: C. 4: B. 5: D. 6: C. 7: B. 8: D. 9: B. 10: C. 11: D. 12: B. 13: C. 14: C. 15: A.

Recipes

Love-Enhancing Recipes by Zola

My All-Time Favorite Homemade Lube

This lube is condom-compatible (you'd better be using them . . . that means you too, Mara Altman!), completely natural, cheap, and, if you go down on your lover, a source of nutritionally valuable essential fatty acids.

The whole world should be as perfect as this recipe.

1 tablespoon of flaxseeds
1 cup of water

Simmer the flaxseeds in the water until the mixture is reduced by half (maybe 20 minutes).

Strain it right away—it gets gooey fast.

If you don't need the lube right away, store it in the fridge. It keeps for up to two weeks in the fridge, but only one to two days at room temperature.

The Tea Trick

At some point during a steamy tryst (preferably when your lover is tied to the bed), step away and make yourself a cup of piping hot tea (milk but no sugar or honey if your lover has a vagina, as these sweeteners feed the yeasty beasties).

Let the tea linger in your mouth so that the heat permeates. Go down (go ahead and be a greedy bitch; use your lover's genitals to make your mouth feel good). When your mouth has cooled down, you can reheat by drinking more tea or take a moment to recite stanzas from Octavio Paz's "Maithuna." . . . Maybe that last one is just my own personal fantasy.

Have fun!

Eric Amaranth on Sex and Eating

I suggest dinner after sex because it always tastes better with afterglow. However, many of us go out to dinner before having sex. Avoid big meals. Eat till you aren't hungry (but not till you feel full). Eat lighter fare like sushi, vegetables, and protein—nothing fried or coated in sauce. Pasta is good for energy if intense sex is to come. If you take a break after an orgasm, lie back with each other and munch on an energy bar and drink some water or have some oranges and bananas.

Pre-Sex Protein Shake

Vanilla protein powder (with no artificial
    sweeteners like aspartame or neotame
    or any other tame)
1 tablespoon cinnamon
2 cups filtered water
2 peaches or 2 bananas
Ice if you like it cold before the hot!

Blend and serve! This keeps you feeling light, but energized.

Orgasm Cookies
by Dr. Barry Komisaruk
(Called "Moon Rocks" by my son Kevin)

This makes more than 150 cookies, necessary to satisfy the demand. However, it is okay to divide recipe by 2 or by 4. Ingredient quantities are not too critical.

4 cups margarine (I use Imperial—nice
    flavor—but you can use butter)
4 cups brown sugar
4 cups white sugar

Blend the above together.

Then blend in:

8 large eggs
4 teaspoons of pure vanilla extract

In separate, *very* large vessel (for full recipe), blend together: ▶

Recipes *(continued)*

4 cups unbleached flour
15 cups quick-cooking oatmeal, raw (yes,
    15 cups—it is just squashed compared to
    regular oatmeal, making it cook quicker;
    it also holds together better in the cookies
    than if you use regular)
2 teaspoons salt
4 teaspoons baking powder
4 teaspoons baking soda
Approximately 72 ounces chocolate chips
    (3 large bags)
Approximately 25 ounces Hershey bars
    (5 large bars, sliced not too thin or small)
Approximately 3 pounds shelled walnuts
    (3 bags)

Mix all ingredients together; will be dense.
    Make golf ball–size cookies. Wet hands
occasionally (batter is sticky).
    I put the raw cookies on a cookie sheet
lined with Reynolds Wrap "Release," which
I think is coated with Teflon. The cookies
don't stick to it. It's not necessary to grease
the "Release," and it can be used repeatedly
for subsequent batches.
    Bake at 375 degrees Fahrenheit
for 10–15 minutes (10 minutes for soft;
13–15 minutes for hard. I prefer hard).
    When I take the baked cookies out of the
oven, I lift the aluminum foil off the cookie
sheets and let the cookies cool on the foil
while I put the next batch of cookies into the
oven on other sheets of foil lining the same
cookie sheets. When the cookies are cool,
they lift off the foil easily and then I reuse the
foil for the next batch. That way cookies are
baking all the time and the baking goes fast.
    This past year, at the request of my son
Adam, I increased the ratio of cookie to
chocolate and nuts, because he complained
that there was too much "stuff" and not

enough "cookie." Others had not voiced such a complaint. Consequently, to even out ratios, you can increase the stuff-to-cookie ratio—not critical. You can also reduce the amount of sugar a bit or use more brown and less white. ◦∿

The Clench and Hold Energy Orgasm, by Barbara Carrellas

BEFORE YOU ACTUALLY START this breathing orgasm, please read through the instructions and then rehearse the individual steps to help your body learn the process.

First, we'll charge the body with breath.

Sit comfortably on the floor.

Relax your jaw.

Yawn. Keep the back of your throat open.

Breathe using the Heart Breath. Breathe in through your mouth using as little effort as possible. Take in as much air as you can with the least possible effort.

Let go. Let the exhale simply fall out. Let it fall out with a sigh. This relaxed little sound will show that you aren't pushing the breath out.

Keep your eyes open. Focus on a point somewhere in the room. You want to stay conscious with your breath and not nod off.

Keep breathing. If you want, you can gently rock back and forth with the breath. You can add Kegels. Make it erotic. Let it feel good. Just remember to stay with the breath.

Set a timer. Breathe for ten minutes—or twenty or thirty! The more you breathe, the more you charge up the body.

When you're ready to do the Clench and Hold, take thirty or so fuller, faster breaths to really charge up.

Lie back on the floor.

Take a full, deep breath. Fill up your lungs from bottom to top. Then let it all go without forcing your breath out.

Take another full, deep breath, and let it go, gently and fully.

Take a third deep breath. Fill up with as

much air as you can hold . . . and . . . hold that breath!

Now here's the important part: As you're holding in your third deep breath, clench every muscle in your body, especially your abdominal muscles, your butt muscles, and your PC muscle. It won't matter much if your hands or your feet aren't clenched, but if your abs, butt, and PC muscle aren't clenched, the Clench and Hold won't be as effective.

There are a number of ways to do this clench.

Lying on your back, you'll want to make sure that you don't put undue stress on your neck or lower back when you tense up, so take a moment and rehearse how you are going to clench before you start breathing. One good way to create the tension you're looking for is to press down into the floor. Try it. Press down into the floor with your hands, shoulders, head, butt, legs, and feet.

Alternatively, extend your body as far as it can go, and reach for opposite walls with your feet and hands.

Or, pull in toward the center of your body as hard as you can—first clench your abs, and then pull the rest of your body in toward your abs.

However you do it, make sure you don't bring your knees up toward your stomach. This releases your abdominal muscles, and that's exactly what you don't want to do!

Keep clenching for about fifteen seconds, and then let go.

Now, here's the hardest part of the Clench and Hold for most people: Have no expectations. Don't try to make anything happen. You have given yourself a huge gift of openness and energy. Just be. ∾

"The Clench and Hold Energy Orgasm" is excerpted from Urban Tantra: Sacred Sex ▶

The Clench and Hold Energy Orgasm
(continued)

Inspirational Things

Inspirational Literature

The Missing Piece Meets the Big O,
  by Shel Silverstein
Fierce Invalids Home from Hot Climates,
  by Tom Robbins
Money, by Martin Amis
What's Your Poo Telling You,
  by Anish Sheth, M.D., and Josh Richman
Breakfast of Champions, by Kurt Vonnegut
Raise High the Roof Beam, Carpenters; and
  Seymour: An Introduction, by J. D. Salinger
One Hundred Years of Solitude,
  by Gabriel García Márquez
Catch-22, by Joseph Heller
Cloud Atlas, by David Mitchell
Woman: An Intimate Geography,
  by Natalie Angier
Women, by Charles Bukowski
The Lorax, by Dr. Seuss
A Confederacy of Dunces,
  by John Kennedy Toole
Shantaram, by Gregory David Roberts
The Savage Detectives, by Roberto Bolaño
Will You Please Be Quiet, Please?,
  by Raymond Carver
Los cuadernos de don Rigoberto,
  by Mario Vargas Llosa

Things That Inspired Me During My Quest

A glass of wine (or three)
Tubs of hummus
Singing "Row, Row, Row Your Boat" in
  rounds with my echo in the shower
Cookies 'n' Cream soft serve (in a cup,
  never a cone)
Salmon sashimi eaten with my hands
Zola's moans
Q-tips
Atman's carrot-raisin scones
Jogging around Prospect Park
Hair in the wrong places ▶

Inspirational Things *(continued)*

Estrella Morente's flamenco music (on repeat
     mode)
The *Lagaan* Bollywood soundtrack (on
     repeat mode)
Bob Marley (on repeat mode)
(okay, almost any song on repeat mode)
Baking anything that has fat-inducing
     properties
Staring at crazy people until I fear they'll
     hurt me
Hank's clit-grinding mound
People who are not too nice, but nice
Having a good MBM—morning bowel
     movement
An iced coffee served with minimal icc (so it
     doesn't get watery) and black so that I can
     have control over my own milk and sugar
     ratios ❧